Checklists for Bartonella, Babesia and Lyme Disease

2012 Edition

J.L. Schaller, M.D., M.A.R. and K. Mountjoy, M.S.

INTERNATIONAL ACADEMIC INFECTION RESEARCH PRESS
Bank Towers • New Gate Center (305)
Highway 41 [Tamiami Trail North]
Naples, FL 34103

Library of Congress Cataloging Data
Schaller, J. L; Mountjoy, K.
Checklists for Bartonella, Babesia and Lyme Disease
by J.L. Schaller and K. Mountjoy

ISBN 978-0-9840889-5-9

1. Tick infections 2. Flea infections 3. Diagnosis

Note on Citation Style

The style of these references varies. Making them uniform would not add to the ability to locate a citation. Most were left as they appeared when uncovered from a wide range of locations.

Manufactured in the United States of America
First Edition

To those working to restore real and concrete liberty to the United States
Specifically, as the world's top jailer, with 25% of the world's
inmates in the USA, we are not the freedom nation,
we are the PRISON NATION.

May God, conscience or peers, help sheriffs, police, child protection
workers, judges and attorney generals to have real integrity,
balance and a heart of service.

In America the abuse of power in law enforcement and child services
is now routine, and character, humility, kindness and wisdom
need to be restored.

If you are working to restore the rights of the poor, weak and falsely
accused—this text and my affection are dedicated to you.

Contents

LYME DISEASE

The Bartonella Checklist

Increasing Suspicion of an Emerging Stealth Infection

James L. Schaller, M.D., M.A.R.

Introduction

In 2011 a new human Bartonella species was added to the over thirty-five Bartonella species currently publically published in Genetic Data banks. It was discovered and highlighted by the talented veterinarian researcher Edward Breitschwerdt. He has said things more clearly than the ideas I was pondering in 2005, while doing most of the research for my Bartonella book. He said simply, but with devastating and highly useful clarity, that **Bartonella testing is terrible, the treatments are poor,** it is typically found on the outside of red blood cells, and the current research on Bartonella is pathetic—one study at NIH. If this was not enough, he said in 2011, **"Bartonella is carried by more vectors than any infection on the earth."** So it is hardly a backdoor "co-infection." Perhaps Lyme is the "co-infection."

Recently, the German researchers Kaiser and Riess summarized Bartonella research in this manner: after 2 decades of Bartonella research, knowledge on transmission and pathology of these bacteria is still limited. Bartonella species have emerged to be important pathogens in human and veterinary medicine.

Why create a check list when a physician can just order an antibody test? First, I have found at times, Bartonella can turn off its own antibodies, and those caused by other tick and flea-borne infections in humans. In a study of sixty-one Bartonella infected dogs, Perez and Maggi reported recently that most Bartonella infected dogs **did not have detectable Bartonella antibodies.**

The criteria listed below may have causes unrelated to Bartonella. For example, each year more studies show the presence of poly infections, and this raises the problem of which infection is causing what symptom, sign or lab test change. For example, most tick infections can cause headache or fatigue. Knowing which infection is the cause does become clear if you are doing very advanced treatments that are designed to kill only one infection. The limitation of these poly infection studies is that typically the testing detection rate for each tick or flea-borne infection is not over 95% for all possible species and strains possibly infecting humans.

However, since Bartonella can disable and kill healthy people, the **checklist below is set to catch virtually every infected patient.** This is neither right nor wrong. Philosophy, sociology, presuppositions, medical fashion and psychology usually all play a role in setting cut offs for a diagnosis. All science is guided by presuppositions, and that is why even math research is guided by a wide range of variables. **In medicine, psychology, philosophical assumptions and sociology control all of medicine** but are unappreciated due to a lack of training. **See Kuhn's** *The Structure of Scientific Revolutions* **exceptionally summarized at the following link: http://des.emory.edu/mfp/Kuhn.html**

THE BARTONELLA CHECKLIST
James Schaller, M.D., M.A.R.
(Please Check Any Symptoms That Apply)

PSYCHIATRIC AND NEUROLOGICAL

☐ Current anxiety that was not present at age ten

☐ Current depression not present at age sixteen

☐ Knee-jerk emotional responses worse than past decades and worsening

☐ Brain fog

☐ Depression

☐ Depression that is not **fully** controlled on **routine anti-depressant doses,** or high dose antidepressants are required to control mood [**Improvement of mood** or being "less depressed" is not successful depression treatment.]

☐ Anxiety is poorly controlled with average dosing

☐ Depression is poorly controlled by reasonable treatment trials.

☐ Suicidal feelings or routine thoughts of death

☐ Crying

☐ Obsessive thoughts or fear in excess of event

☐ Obsessive thoughts that intrude into the mind which are in excess of normal

☐ A decrease in pleasure

☐ Rage worse with time

☐ Irritability worse with time

☐ Impatience is greater when compared to ten years ago [in a child--any irritability in excess of what is common for most children with an identical age].

☐ Cursing or hostile speech that is worse over time

☐ Increased addictions that are very resistant to typical recovery ranges

☐ Increased impulsivity in contrast to past years or past decades

☐ Severe neurological disorders without a clear cause

☐ Severe psychiatric troubles that do not seem to fit with the diagnostic criteria or there is trouble controlling symptoms with treatment

☐ New physical, emotional or verbal abuse in the home which was not present in the past

☐ Panic attacks that were not present at ten years of age

☐ Anxiety medication has to be increased to **very high levels** to continue past benefit

☐ Diagnosed as having bipolar disorder, but do not fit the criteria well

☐ Any psychiatric disorder that also shows **medical pathology in laboratory tests**

☐ Restlessness

☐ Combative behavior

☐ A parent, grandparent, child or sibling with suicide attempts

☐ A parent, grandparent, child or sibling who has started physical or extreme verbal fights

☐ Intermittent confusion

☐ Seizures

☐ Brain lesions seen on a brain scan such as an MRI or CT of the head

☐ Short term memory deficits

☐ Difficulty in learning new information

DERMATOLOGY OR SKIN

☐ Persistent rashes that last over 3 weeks

☐ Nodules under the skin

☐ Hyper-pigmentation or dark areas of skin which were not present at birth

☐ Hypo-pigmentation or obvious light areas of skin

☐ Unexplained hair loss

☐ Spontaneous breaks or holes in the skin as small as a millimeter

☐ Skin ulcerations

☐ Stretch marks in eccentric locations, e.g., arms, upper side under armpit, around armpit or on the back

☐ Stretch marks filled with red, pink, purple or dark blue color which are not caused by pregnancy or weight loss [remember, many with many pregnancies or weight loss do not have 20 stretch marks]

☐ Any skin markings or growths **greater** than most people

☐ Blood vessels or color on skin **greater** than most people

☐ Red papules of **any** size

☐ Skin tags including ones removed by a dermatologist or shaved off

☐ Unusual blood vessels of any kind including inside organs such as bladder or intestinal walls

☐ Any skin finding in excess of 95% of most humans

☐ Skin findings showing increased blood vessels of any size

☐ Skin findings showing increased tissue formation that is increased over the flatness of surface skin [This may be due to Bartonella, untreated Lyme disease, or both infections and systemic inflammation]

☐ Skin showing blood vessels that are too large or too many for **the location of the blood vessels**, e.g., surface thigh and calf skin with very thick surface blood vessels or legs, upper arms or shoulders have explosions of many fine blood vessels

☐ Burning skin sensations [this may have many causes].

☐ Itching without a clear cause and which is hard to control and remove

☐ Skin erosion without a clear cause such as a fire, fall or chemical burn

☐ Minor cuts or scratches which heal slowly

☐ Very slow healing after a surgery

☐ "Granulomas" or balls of tissue

☐ Formication or feelings of being bitten by bugs or bug sensations on skin with no bugs on the skin

EYE

☐ Retina infection

☐ Retina infarct or dead tissue in the back of the eye

☐ Neuroretinitis or inflammation of the retina and optic nerve in the back of the eye

☐ Uveitis or inflammation of the middle layer of the eye or the interior eye

☐ Papilledema or swelling of the optic nerve as it enters the back of the eye due to raised intracranial pressure

☐ Stellate maculopathy

☐ Acute blurred vision

☐ Sudden and/or significant change in vision

HEART

☐ Endocarditis or inflammation of the heart

☐ Heart valve pathology

☐ Enlargement of the heart

☐ Any amount of dead cardiac tissue

☐ Arrhythmias of the heart

☐ Palpitations unrelated to panic attacks

GENERAL MEDICAL

☐ Sleep medications take 90-120 minute to take effect instead of 30 minutes

☐ Insomnia [If profound fatigue is present, this might not apply]

☐ A temperature under 98.3 in a sick person.   A temperature under 99.0 if Lyme disease or Babesia is also present

☐ An uncomfortable infection in the body with no discernible cause

☐ Gastroesophageal reflux disease (GERD)

☐ Diarrhea

☐ Colitis or an inflammation of the colon

☐ Liver enlargement with no clear cause

☐ Blood vessel proliferation or increased numbers in any internal organs

☐ Lesions or wounds with no clear cause

☐ A sore throat with no other clear reason

☐ A persistent sore throat in humidity in excess of 45% [low humidity dries out throat tissue]

☐ Gingivitis or bleeding during flossing

☐ Unusual discomfort on the soles of the feet especially in the morning

☐ Puffy tissue on insole or any part of ankles

☐ Ankle "edema" or expanded tissue that does not pit when pressed [because it is expanded tissue and not merely fluid]

☐ Bone pain

☐ Inflammation of the outer bone surface or osteomyelitis

☐ Joint pain [this can be also due to Lyme disease and many other medical problems]

☐ Muscle pain [this can be also due to Lyme disease and many other medical problems]

☐ Medical problems described as "idiopathic" (of unknown or unclear cause)

☐ Presence of two tick or flea infections with two positive tick or flea-borne viruses, bacteria or protozoa.

As previously mentioned, Bartonella has more than 30 published species in public genetic databases and has more vectors than possibly any infection in the world. Therefore, the presence of other infections such as tick-borne viruses, bacteria or protozoa, should raise suspicion. Some of these include Babesia, STARI (Masterson's Disease), Neoehrlichia, Anaplasma, Lyme disease, Mycoplasmas, Q Fever, Rocky Mountain spotted fever (Rickettsia), tick-borne relapsing fever, Tularemia (bacteria), Ehrlichia, Protozoa FL1953, and viruses such as CMV, HHV-6, Coxsackie B Types 1, 2, 3, 4, 5, 6, Parvo B-19 or Powassan.

POSSIBLE LABORATORY FINDINGS

☐ IL-6 is very low.

☐ IL-1B is very low.

☐ TNF-alpha is in lower 10% of normal range.

☐ VEGF is above the normal range [however, if Babesia is present or being treated the VEGF will fall into normal or abnormal low levels].

☐ X-ray of the bone may show areas of bone loss.

☐ Biopsies of lymph nodes are negative for Mycoplasma and no clear evidence of other infections or illnesses are found

☐ Biopsies of lymph nodes appearing similar to sarcoidosis

☐ Tissue biopsies which are abnormal but with no clear cause of tissue problems

☐ A swab of a fresh scratch or bite skin lesion is positive for Bartonella.

ENVIRONMENT

☐ Exposure to cats and dogs in excess of very incidental rare contact

☐ **Exposure to cats and dogs** that have been strays or go outside [reviews of hundreds of professional journal articles make this a risk in an unknown percentage]

☐ Ticks or fleas are found on any pet you contact

☐ The patient's **mother** is suspected of having Bartonella based on newer direct and **indirect testing.**

☐ A **sibling, father, spouse or child** with any tick or flea-borne infection who shared with the patient a residence or vacation location with proximity to brush

☐ Outdoor exposure to outdoor environments such as brush, wild grasses, wild streams or woods which happened **without** the use of DEET on skin and Permethrin on all clothing (**It only takes one exposure to get a bite**. If you used protection "most of the time," you were still exposed.)

☐ Exposure to lice

☐ Flea bites or flea exposure

☐ Exposure to pets that are exposed to ticks or fleas

☐ A scratch from a cat

☐ A bite from a cat or dog

☐ Exposure to biting flies

☐ Hunting, living or vacationing near deer or small mammals

☐   Clear exposure to any type of tick. [Bartonella is carried by
     a huge number of carriers, but for now, the percent that carry
     Bartonella is not known.   Further, the capacity to detect all new
     species in the vectors or in humans infected does not exist or is
     not routinely available in direct testing of all human infectious
     Bartonella organisms in both large or specialty labs].

☐   Ticks found on your clothing

☐   Ticks found on your skin

☐   Ticks found in your home or car, vacation spot or recreation area

If one reads the majority of Bartonella journal articles, it seems clear
Bartonella harms the body in hundreds of ways. But for our purposes
in diagnosis, the above criteria should be enough to prevent a missed
diagnosis. More criteria exist. Certainty claims or criticism about
Bartonella positions without reading at least of 1,000 articles is confusing.
How is this possible with new Bartonella findings and understandings
each month? There are also new species whose genetic sequences show
their uniqueness almost every month in public databases. In this spirit,
this scale is meant merely to increase suspicion of Bartonella, which is a
super stealth infection that takes perhaps fifty days to grow out on some
bacteria growth plates, and floats in the blood as it lowers fevers. It also
clearly suppresses some key immune system fighting chemicals. Cure
claims made without the use of **indirect** testing, markedly documented
in superior journals, should be examined further to prove effectiveness.

**Dr. Schaller is the author of 30 books and 27 top journal articles.
His publications address issues in at least twelve fields of medicine.
He has the most recent textbook on Bartonella. He has published on
Bartonella under the supervision of the former editor of the *Journal
of the American Medical Association (JAMA)*, and his entries on
multiple tick and flea borne infections, including Bartonella [along
with Babesia and Lyme disease] were published in a respected
infection textbook endorsed by the NIH Director of Infectious
Disease.   He has seven texts on tick and flea-borne infections based
on his markedly unique full-time research and study practice, which
is not limited to either finite traditional or integrative progressive**

medicine. Dr. Schaller has read on these emerging problems for many years.

Bibliography (Bartonella)

Aberer E. Lyme borreliosis--an update. J Dtsch Dermatol Ges. 2007 May;5(5):406-14. [Article in English, German]. J Dtsch Dermatol Ges. 2007 May;5(5):406-14. PMID:17451386

Abuzeid WM, Ruckenstein MJ. Spirochetes in otology: are we testing for the right pathogens?   Otolaryngol Head Neck Surg. 2008 Jan;138(1):107-9. PMID:18165003

Accorinti M. Ocular bartonellosis. Int J Med Sci. 2009;6(3):131-2. Epub 2009 Mar 19. PMID:19319232

Adamska M. [Bartonella spp. as a zoonotic pathogens transmitting by blood-feeding arthropods].[Article in Polish]. Wiad Parazytol. 2010;56(1):1-9. PMID:20450002

Aguero-Rosenfeld ME, Wang G, Schwartz I, Wormser GP. Diagnosis of lyme borreliosis. Clin Microbiol Rev. 2005 Jul;18(3):484-509. PMID:16020686

Al-Attar N, Ruimy R, Baron F, Hvass U. Bartonella endocarditis complicating congenital heart disease. BMJ Case Rep. 2009;2009. pii: bcr06.2008.0092. Epub 2009 Mar 17. PMID:21686936

Alves AS, Milhano N, Santos-Silva M, Santos AS, Vilhena M, de Sousa R. Evidence of Bartonella spp., Rickettsia spp. and Anaplasma phagocytophilum in domestic, shelter and stray cat blood and fleas, Portugal. Clin Microbiol Infect. 2009 Dec;15 Suppl 2:1-3. Epub 2009 Mar 26. PMID:19416279

Anan'eva LP, Studentsov EE, Levin E. [Detection of anti-Borrelia antibodies by immunoblotting in Lyme borreliosis].[Article in Russian]. Klin Lab Diagn. 2002 Jun;(6):45-7. PMID:12132378

Ang CW, Notermans DW, Hommes M, Simoons-Smit AM, Herremans T. Large differences between test strategies for the detection of anti-Borrelia antibodies are revealed by comparing eight ELISAs and five immunoblots. Eur J Clin Microbiol Infect Dis. 2011 Aug;30(8):1027-32. Epub 2011 Jan 27. PMID:21271270

Angelakis E, Edouard S, La Scola B, Raoult D. Bartonella henselae in skin biopsy specimens of patients with cat-scratch disease. Emerg Infect Dis. 2010 Dec;16(12):1963-5. PMID:21122232

Angelakis E, Lepidi H, Canel A, Rispal P, Perraudeau F, Barre I, Rolain JM, Raoult D. Human case of Bartonella alsatica lymphadenitis. Emerg Infect Dis. 2008 Dec;14(12):1951-3. PMID:19046532

Angelakis E, Pulcini C, Waton J, Imbert P, Socolovschi C, Edouard S, Dellamonica P, Raoult D. Scalp eschar and neck lymphadenopathy caused by Bartonella henselae after Tick Bite. Clin Infect Dis. 2010 Feb 15;50(4):549-51. PMID:20070235

Angelakis E, Roux V, Raoult D, Rolain JM. Real-time PCR strategy and detection of bacterial agents of lymphadenitis. Eur J Clin Microbiol Infect Dis. 2009 Nov;28(11):1363-8. Epub 2009 Aug 14. PMID:19685089

Arav-Boger R, Crawford T, Steere AC, Halsey NA. Cerebellar ataxia as the presenting manifestation of Lyme disease. Pediatr Infect Dis J. 2002 Apr;21(4):353-6. PMID:12075773

Arvand M, Raoult D, Feil EJ. Multi-locus sequence typing of a geographically and temporally diverse sample of the highly clonal human pathogen Bartonella quintana. PLoS One. 2010 Mar 19;5(3):e9765. PMID:20333257

Assi MA, Yao JD, Walker RC. Lyme disease followed by human granulocytic anaplasmosis in a kidney transplant recipient. Transpl Infect Dis. 2007 Mar;9(1):66-72. PMID:17313478

Atamanyuk I, Raja SG, Kostolny M. Bartonella henselae endocarditis of percutaneously implanted pulmonary valve: a case report. J Heart Valve Dis. 2011 Jan;20(1):94-7. PMID:21396492

Bacon RM, Biggerstaff BJ, Schriefer ME, Gilmore RD Jr, Philipp MT, Steere AC, Wormser GP, Marques AR, Johnson BJ. Serodiagnosis of Lyme disease by kinetic enzyme-linked immunosorbent assay using recombinant VlsE1 or peptide antigens of Borrelia burgdorferi compared with 2-tiered testing using whole-cell lysates. J Infect Dis. 2003 Apr 15;187(8):1187-99. Epub 2003 Apr 2. PMID:12695997

Bakken JS, Dumler JS. Clinical diagnosis and treatment of human granulocytotropic anaplasmosis. Ann N Y Acad Sci. 2006 Oct;1078:236-47. PMID:17114714

Ball R, Shadomy SV, Meyer A, Huber BT, Leffell MS, Zachary A, Belotto M, Hilton E, Bryant-Genevier M, Schriefer ME, Miller FW, Braun MM. HLA type and immune response to Borrelia burgdorferi outer surface protein a in people in whom arthritis developed after Lyme disease vaccination. Arthritis Rheum. 2009 Apr;60(4):1179-86. PMID:19333928

Barbier F, Fournier PE, Dauge MC, Gallien S, Raoult D, Andremont A, Ruimy R. Bartonella quintana coinfection in Staphylococcus aureus endocarditis: usefulness of screening in high-risk patients? Clin Infect Dis. 2009 May 1;48(9):1332-3. PMID:19344260

Baty G, Lanotte P, Hocqueloux L, Prazuck T, Bret L, Romano M, Mereghetti L. [PCR rDNA 16S used for the etiological diagnosis of blood culture negative endocarditis].[Article in French]. Med Mal Infect. 2010 Jun;40(6):358-62. Epub 2009 Sep 30. PMID:19796889

Bayliss DB, Steiner JM, Sucholdolski JS, Radecki SV, Brewer MM, Morris AK, Lappin MR. Serum feline pancreatic lipase immunoreactivity concentration and seroprevalences of antibodies against Toxoplasma gondii and Bartonella species in client-owned cats. J Feline Med Surg. 2009 Aug;11(8):663-7. Epub 2009 Jun 26. PMID:19560385

Beall MJ, Chandrashekar R, Eberts MD, Cyr KE, Diniz PP, Mainville C, Hegarty BC, Crawford JM, Breitschwerdt EB. Serological and molecular prevalence of Borrelia burgdorferi, Anaplasma phagocytophilum, and Ehrlichia species in dogs from Minnesota. Vector Borne Zoonotic Dis. 2008 Aug;8(4):455-64. PMID:18302532

Becker JL. Vector-borne illnesses and the safety of the blood supply. Curr Hematol Rep. 2003 Nov;2(6):511-7. PMID:14561396

Belgard S, Truyen U, Thibault JC, Sauter-Louis C, Hartmann K. Relevance of feline calicivirus, feline immunodeficiency virus, feline leukemia virus, feline herpesvirus and Bartonella henselae in cats with chronic gingivostomatitis. Berl Munch Tierarztl Wochenschr. 2010 Sep-Oct;123(9-10):369-76. PMID:21038808

Bellissimo-Rodrigues F, da Fonseca BA, Martinez R. Bacillary angiomatosis in a pregnant woman. Int J Gynaecol Obstet. 2010 Oct;111(1):85-6. Epub 2010 Jul 21. PMID:20650456

Bernabeu-Wittel J, Luque R, Corbi R, Mantrana-Bermejo M, Navarrete M, Vallejo A, Bernabeu-Wittel M. Bacillary angiomatosis with atypical clinical presentation in an immunocompetent patient. Indian J Dermatol Venereol Leprol. 2010 Nov-Dec;76(6):682-5. PMID:21079313

Bhengsri S, Baggett HC, Peruski LF Jr, Morway C, Bai Y, Fisk TL, Sitdhirasdr A, Maloney SA, Dowell SF, Kosoy M. Bartonella spp. infections, Thailand. Emerg Infect Dis. 2010 Apr;16(4):743-5. PMID:20350414

Bhengsri S, Baggett HC, Peruski LF, Morway C, Bai Y, Fisk TL, Sitdhirasdr A, Maloney SA, Dowell SF, Kosoy M. Bartonella seroprevalence in rural Thailand. Southeast Asian J Trop Med Public Health. 2011 May;42(3):687-92. PMID:21706948

Bhide M, Yilmaz Z, Golcu E, Torun S, Mikula I. Seroprevalence of anti-Borrelia burgdorferi antibodies in dogs and horses in Turkey. Ann Agric Environ Med. 2008 Jun;15(1):85-90. PMID:18581984

Bianda JC, Dedes W. [Positive polymerase chain reaction for Bartonella henselae in conjunctival granuloma].[Article in German]. Klin Monbl Augenheilkd. 2009 Apr;226(4):347. Epub 2009 Apr 21. PMID:19384797

Binnicker MJ, Jespersen DJ, Harring JA, Rollins LO, Bryant SC, Beito EM. Evaluation of two commercial systems for automated processing, reading, and interpretation of Lyme borreliosis Western blots. J Clin Microbiol. 2008 Jul;46(7):2216-21. Epub 2008 May 7. PMID:18463211

Bitam I, Dittmar K, Parola P, Whiting MF, Raoult D. Fleas and flea-borne diseases. Int J Infect Dis. 2010 Aug;14(8):e667-76. Epub 2010 Mar 1. PMID:20189862

Blanco JR, Jado I, Marín M, Sanfeliu I, Portillo A, Anda P, Pons I, Oteo JA. [Microbiological diagnosis of emerging bacterial pathogens: Anaplasma, Bartonella, Rickettsia, and Tropheryma whipplei].[Article in Spanish]. Enferm Infecc Microbiol Clin. 2008 Nov;26(9):573-80. PMID:19100178

Bodaghi B. [New etiological concepts in uveitis].[Article in French]. J Fr Ophtalmol. 2005 May;28(5):547-55. PMID:15976725

Bodaghi B. [Ocular manifestations of Lyme disease].[Article in French]. Med Mal Infect. 2007 Jul-Aug;37(7-8):518-22. Epub 2007 Mar 21. PMID:17376626

Boggs SR, Fisher RG. Bone pain and fever in an adolescent and his sibling. Cat scratch disease (CSD). Pediatr Infect Dis J. 2011 Jan;30(1):89, 93-4. PMID:21513084

Bolton JG, Galeckas KJ, Satter EK. Inoculation bartonellosis in an adult: a case report. Cutis. 2010 Jan;85(1):37-42. PMID:20184210

Boltri JM, Hash RB, Vogel RL. Patterns of Lyme disease diagnosis and treatment by family physicians in a southeastern state. J Community Health. 2002 Dec;27(6):395-402. PMID:12458782

Branda JA, Aguero-Rosenfeld ME, Ferraro MJ, Johnson BJ, Wormser GP, Steere AC. 2-tiered antibody testing for early and late Lyme disease using only an immunoglobulin G blot with the addition of a VlsE band as the second-tier test. Clin Infect Dis. 2010 Jan 1;50(1):20-6. PMID:19947857

Branda JA, Linskey K, Kim YA, Steere AC, Ferraro MJ. Two-tiered antibody testing for Lyme disease with use of 2 enzyme immunoassays, a whole-cell sonicate enzyme immunoassay followed by a VlsE C6 peptide enzyme immunoassay. Clin Infect Dis. 2011 Sep;53(6):541-7. PMID:21865190

Breitschwerdt EB, Maggi RG. A confusing case of canine vector-borne disease: clinical signs and progression in a dog co-infected with Ehrlichia canis and Bartonella vinsonii ssp, berkhoffii. Parasit Vectors. 2009 Mar 26;2 Suppl 1:S3. PMID:19426442

Breitschwerdt EB, Maggi RG. Comparative medical features of canine and human bartonellosis. Clin Microbiol Infect. 2009 Dec;15 Suppl 2:106-7. Epub 2009 Apr 30. PMID:19438635

Breitschwerdt EB, Maggi RG, Varanat M, Linder KE, Weinberg G. Isolation of Bartonella vinsonii subsp. berkhoffii genotype II from a boy with epithelioid hemangioendothelioma and a dog with hemangiopericytoma. J Clin Microbiol. 2009 Jun;47(6):1957-60. Epub 2009 Apr 15. PMID:19369441

Brewer NT, Weinstein ND, Cuite CL, Herrington JE. Risk perceptions and their relation to risk behavior. Ann Behav Med. 2004 Apr;27(2):125-30. PMID:15026296

Brinar VV, Habek M. Rare infections mimicking MS. Clin Neurol Neurosurg. 2010 Sep;112(7):625-8. Epub 2010 May 2. PMID:20439131

Brook I. The bacteriology of salivary gland infections. Oral Maxillofac Surg Clin North Am. 2009 Aug;21(3):269-74. PMID:19608044

Brown DB, Huang YC, Kannenberg EL, Sherrier DJ, Carlson RW. An acpXL mutant of Rhizobium leguminosarum bv. phaseoli lacks 27-hydroxyoctacosanoic acid in its lipid A and is developmentally delayed during symbiotic infection of the determinate nodulating host plant Phaseolus vulgaris. J Bacteriol. 2011 Sep;193(18):4766-78. Epub 2011 Jul 15. PMID:21764936

Brown EL, Kim JH, Reisenbichler ES, Höök M. Multicomponent Lyme vaccine: three is not a crowd. Vaccine. 2005 May 25;23(28):3687-96. PMID:15882529

Buchmann AU, Kempf VA, Kershaw O, Gruber AD. Peliosis hepatis in cats is not associated with Bartonella henselae infections. Vet Pathol. 2010 Jan;47(1):163-6. PMID:20080497

Bunikis J, Barbour AG. Laboratory testing for suspected Lyme disease. Med Clin North Am. 2002 Mar;86(2):311-40. PMID:11982304

Burbelo PD, Bren KE, Ching KH, Coleman A, Yang X, Kariu T, Iadarola MJ, Pal U. Antibody profiling of Borrelia burgdorferi infection in horses. Clin Vaccine Immunol. 2011 Sep;18(9):1562-7. Epub 2011 Jul 20. PMID:21775514

Capitta P, Zobba R, Masala G, Cocco R, Tola S, Parpaglia ML. Isolation and characterization of Bartonella strains in cats in Italy. Transbound Emerg Dis. 2010 Jun;57(3):201-4. Epub 2010 Mar 14. PMID:20345572

Caponetti GC, Pantanowitz L, Marconi S, Havens JM, Lamps LW, Otis CN. Evaluation of immunohistochemistry in identifying Bartonella henselae in cat-scratch disease. Am J Clin Pathol. 2009 Feb;131(2):250-6. PMID:19141385

Carvounis PE, Mehta AP, Geist CE. Orbital myositis associated with Borrelia burgdorferi (Lyme disease) infection. Ophthalmology. 2004 May;111(5):1023-8. PMID:15121383

Casalta JP, Gouriet F, Richet H, Thuny F, Habib G, Raoult
D. Prevalence of Coxiella burnetii and Bartonella species as
cases of infective endocarditis in Marseilles (1994-2007). Clin
Microbiol Infect. 2009 Dec;15 Suppl 2:152-3. Epub 2009 Sep 28.
PMID:19793124

Cermakova Z, Ryskova O, Honegr K, Cermakova E, Hanovcova I.
Diagnosis of Lyme borreliosis using enzyme immunoanalysis. Med Sci
Monit. 2005 Apr;11(4):BR121-5. Epub 2005 Mar 24. PMID:15795690

Cetin E, Sotoudeh M, Auer H, Stanek G. Paradigm Burgenland: risk
of Borrelia burgdorferi sensu lato infection indicated by variable
seroprevalence rates in hunters. Wien Klin Wochenschr. 2006
Nov;118(21-22):677-81. PMID:17160606

Chang CC, Chen YJ, Tseng CS, Lai WL, Hsu KY, Chang CL, Lu
CC, Hsu YM. A comparative study of the interaction of Bartonella
henselae strains with human endothelial cells. Vet Microbiol. 2011 Apr
21;149(1-2):147-56. Epub 2010 Oct 7. PMID:21035278

Cherry NA, Maggi RG, Cannedy AL, Breitschwerdt EB. PCR
detection of Bartonella bovis and Bartonella henselae in the blood of
beef cattle. Vet Microbiol. 2009 Mar 30;135(3-4):308-12. Epub 2008
Sep 21. PMID:19019574

Cheung VW, Moxham JP. Cat scratch disease presenting as acute
mastoiditis. Laryngoscope. 2010;120 Suppl 4:S222. PMID:21225820

Chiaraviglio L, Duong S, Brown DA, Birtles RJ, Kirby JE. An
immunocompromised murine model of chronic Bartonella infection.
Am J Pathol. 2010 Jun;176(6):2753-63. Epub 2010 Apr 15.
PMID:20395436

Chmielewski T, Fiett J, Gniadkowski M, Tylewska-Wierzbanowska
S. Improvement in the laboratory recognition of lyme borreliosis with
the combination of culture and PCR methods. Mol Diagn. 2003;7(3-
4):155-62. PMID:15068385

Choi P, Qin X, Chen EY, Inglis AF Jr, Ou HC, Perkins JA, Sie KC, Patterson K, Berry S, Manning SC. Polymerase chain reaction for pathogen identification in persistent pediatric cervical lymphadenitis. Arch Otolaryngol Head Neck Surg. 2009 Mar;135(3):243-8. PMID:19289701

Chomel BB, Kasten RW, Williams C, Wey AC, Henn JB, Maggi R, Carrasco S, Mazet J, Boulouis HJ, Maillard R, Breitschwerdt EB. Bartonella endocarditis: a pathology shared by animal reservoirs and patients. Ann N Y Acad Sci. 2009 May;1166:120-6. PMID:19538271

Chu BC, Tam VT. A serologically proven case of cat-scratch disease presenting with neuroretinitis. Hong Kong Med J. 2009 Oct;15(5):391-3. PMID:19801700

Colton L, Zeidner N, Lynch T, Kosoy MY. Human isolates of Bartonella tamiae induce pathology in experimentally inoculated immunocompetent mice. BMC Infect Dis. 2010 Jul 30;10:229. PMID:20673363

Coulter P, Lema C, Flayhart D, Linhardt AS, Aucott JN, Auwaerter PG, Dumler JS. Two-year evaluation of Borrelia burgdorferi culture and supplemental tests for definitive diagnosis of Lyme disease. J Clin Microbiol. 2005 Oct;43(10):5080-4. PMID:16207966

Costa V, Sommese L, Casamassimi A, Colicchio R, Angelini C, Marchesano V, Milone L, Farzati B, Giovane A, Fiorito C, Rienzo M, Picardi M, Avallone B, Marco Corsi M, Sarubbi B, Calabrò R, Salvatore P, Ciccodicola A, Napoli C. Impairment of circulating endothelial progenitors in Down syndrome. BMC Med Genomics. 2010 Sep 13;3:40. PMID:20836844

Coyle PK. Lyme disease. Curr Neurol Neurosci Rep. 2002 Nov;2(6):479-87. PMID:12359100

Cunha BA, Cohen YZ, McDermott B. Fever of unknown origin (FUO) due to babesiosis in a immunocompetent host. Heart Lung. 2008 Nov-Dec;37(6):481-4. Epub 2008 Sep 30. PMID:18992633

Curi AL, Machado D, Heringer G, Campos WR, Lamas C, Rozental T, Gutierres A, Orefice F, Lemos E. Cat-scratch disease: ocular manifestations and visual outcome. Int Ophthalmol. 2010 Oct;30(5):553-8. Epub 2010 Jul 30. PMID:20668914

Da Silva K, Chussid S. Cat scratch disease: clinical considerations for the pediatric dentist. Pediatr Dent. 2009 Jan-Feb;31(1):58-62. PMID:19320261

Dabrowska-Bień J, Pietniczka-Załeska M, Rowicki T. [Cat scratch disease--a diagnostic problem, case report].[Article in Polish]. Otolaryngol Pol. 2009 Mar-Apr;63(2):154-7. PMID:19681487

Das BB, Wasser E, Bryant KA, Woods CR, Yang SG, Zahn M. Culture negative endocarditis caused by Bartonella henselae in a child with congenital heart disease. Pediatr Infect Dis J. 2009 Oct;28(10):922-5. PMID:19738506

Dautović-Krkić S, Cavaljuga S, Ferhatović M, Mostarac N, Gojak R, Hadzović M, Hadzić A. [Lyme borreliosis in Bosnia and Herzegovina--clinical, laboratory and epidemiological research].[Article in Bosnian]. Med Arh. 2008;62(2):107-10. PMID:18669233

de Caprariis D, Dantas-Torres F, Capelli G, Mencke N, Stanneck D, Breitschwerdt EB, Otranto D. Evolution of clinical, haematological and biochemical findings in young dogs naturally infected by vector-borne pathogens. Vet Microbiol. 2011 Apr 21;149(1-2):206-12. Epub 2010 Oct 16. PMID:21106311

de La Blanchardière A, Fournier PE, Haustraete E, du Cheyron D, Lepage O, Verdon R. [Infective endocarditis due to Bartonella henselae following a rupture of a cerebral aneurysm].[Article in French]. Med Mal Infect. 2009 Jun;39(6):394-6. Epub 2008 Dec 18. PMID:19097835

De Martino SJ. [Role of biological assays in the diagnosis of Lyme borreliosis presentations. What are the techniques and which are currently available?].[Article in French]. Med Mal Infect. 2007 Jul-Aug;37(7-8):496-506. Epub 2007 May 23. PMID:17512148

De Martino S, Jaulhac B. [Lyme borreliosis].[Article in French]. Rev Prat. 2005 Mar 15;55(5):471-7. PMID:15895947

de Paz HD, Larrea D, Zunzunegui S, Dehio C, de la Cruz F, Llosa M. Functional dissection of the conjugative coupling protein TrwB. J Bacteriol. 2010 Jun;192(11):2655-69. Epub 2010 Apr 2. PMID:20363945

Dekkers MJ, Dees A, Weidema WF, Bartelsman M, Veeken H, Hart W. [Clinical thinking and decision making in practice. A man with abdominal pain, weight loss and fever].[Article in Dutch]. Ned Tijdschr Geneeskd. 2009 Jan 31;153(5):174-80. PMID:19256242

Delforge ML. [On the usefulness of serology testing in infectious diseases: selected topics].[Article in French]. Rev Med Brux. 2011 Sep;32(4):285-8. PMID:22034758

DePietropaolo DL, Powers JH, Gill JM, Foy AJ. Diagnosis of lyme disease. Am Fam Physician. 2005 Jul 15;72(2):297-304. PMID:16050454

DePietropaolo DL, Powers JH, Gill JM, Foy AJ. Diagnosis of Lyme disease. Del Med J. 2006 Jan;78(1):11-8. PMID:16548394

Desenclos JC, Laporte A, Brouqui P. [Louse-borne infections in humans].[Article in French]. Med Mal Infect. 2011 Jun;41(6):295-300. Epub 2011 Mar 30. PMID:21450425

Dessau RB, Bangsborg JM, Ejlertsen T, Skarphedinsson S, Schønheyder HC. Utilization of serology for the diagnosis of suspected Lyme borreliosis in Denmark: survey of patients seen in general practice. BMC Infect Dis. 2010 Nov 1;10:317. PMID:21040576

Dessau RB, Bangsborg JM, Jensen TP, Hansen K, Lebech AM, Andersen CØ. [Laboratory diagnosis of infection caused by Borrelia burgdorferi].[Article in Danish]. Ugeskr Laeger. 2006 Aug 21;168(34):2805-7. PMID:16942701

Diniz PP, Wood M, Maggi RG, Sontakke S, Stepnik M, Breitschwerdt EB. Co-isolation of Bartonella henselae and Bartonella vinsonii subsp. Berkhoffii from blood, joint and subcutaneous seroma fluids from two naturally infected dogs. Vet Microbiol. 2009 Sep 18;138(3-4):368-72. Epub 2009 Feb 4. PMID:19560291

Donnelly EF. Preview: Lyme disease vaccines. Med Health R I. 1998 Nov;81(11):373-5. PMID:15580796

dos Santos AP, dos Santos RP, Biondo AW, Dora JM, Goldani LZ, de Oliveira ST, de Sá Guimarães AM, Timenetsky J, de Morais HA, González FH, Messick JB. Hemoplasma infection in HIV-positive patient, Brazil. Emerg Infect Dis. 2008 Dec;14(12):1922-4. PMID:19046522

Douglas TA, Tamburro D, Fredolini C, Espina BH, Lepene BS, Ilag L, Espina V, Petricoin EF 3rd, Liotta LA, Luchini A. The use of hydrogel microparticles to sequester and concentrate bacterial antigens in a urine test for Lyme disease. Biomaterials. 2011 Feb;32(4):1157-66. Epub 2010 Oct 28. PMID:21035184

Dowers KL, Hawley JR, Brewer MM, Morris AK, Radecki SV, Lappin MR. Association of Bartonella species, feline calicivirus, and feline herpesvirus 1 infection with gingivostomatitis in cats. J Feline Med Surg. 2010 Apr;12(4):314-21. Epub 2009 Dec 2. PMID:19959386

Drummond MR, Gilioli R, Velho PE. Bartonellosis diagnosis requires careful evaluation. Braz J Infect Dis. 2010 May-Jun;14(3):217. PMID:20835501

Dubey JP, Bhatia CR, Lappin MR, Ferreira LR, Thorn A, Kwok OC. Seroprevalence of Toxoplasma gondii and Bartonella spp. antibodies in cats from Pennsylvania. J Parasitol. 2009 Jun;95(3):578-80. PMID:19061304

Dubey JP, Lappin MR, Kwok OC, Mofya S, Chikweto A, Baffa A, Doherty D, Shakeri J, Macpherson CN, Sharma RN. Seroprevalence of Toxoplasma gondii and concurrent Bartonella spp., feline immunodeficiency virus, and feline leukemia virus infections in cats from Grenada, West Indies. J Parasitol. 2009 Oct;95(5):1129-33. Epub 2009 Apr 22. PMID:19385716

Durá-Travé T, Yoldi-Petri ME, Gallinas-Victoriano F, Lavilla-Oiz A, Bove-Guri M. Neuroretinitis Caused by Bartonella henselae (Cat-Scratch Disease) in a 13-Year-Old Girl. Int J Pediatr. 2010;2010:763105. Epub 2010 Jun 15. PMID:20628521

Dutta A, Schwarzwald HL, Edwards MS. Disseminated bartonellosis presenting as neuroretinitis in a young adult with human immunodeficiency virus infection. Pediatr Infect Dis J. 2010 Jul;29(7):675-7. PMID:20216243

Edlow JA. Erythema migrans. Med Clin North Am. 2002 Mar;86(2):239-60. PMID:11982300

Edouard S, Gonin K, Turc Y, Angelakis E, Socolovschi C, Raoult D. Eschar and neck lymphadenopathy caused by Francisella tularensis after a tick bite: a case report. J Med Case Reports. 2011 Mar 19;5:108. PMID:21418587

Edouard S, Raoult D. [Bartonella henselae, an ubiquitous agent of proteiform zoonotic disease].[Article in French]. Med Mal Infect. 2010 Jun;40(6):319-30. Epub 2009 Dec 29. PMID:20042306

Eisen L, Eisen RJ, Chang CC, Mun J, Lane RS. Acarologic risk of exposure to Borrelia burgdorferi spirochaetes: long-term evaluations in north-western California, with implications for Lyme borreliosis risk-assessment models. Med Vet Entomol. 2004 Mar;18(1):38-49. PMID:15009444

Eldøen G, Vik IS, Vik E, Midgard R. [Lyme neuroborreliosis in More and Romsdal].[Article in Norwegian]. Tidsskr Nor Laegeforen. 2001 Jun 30;121(17):2008-11. PMID:11875896

Elston DM, Do H. What's eating you? Cat flea (Ctenocephalides felis), Part 1: Clinical features and role as a disease vector. Cutis. 2010 May;85(5):231-6. PMID:20540412

Eppes SC, Childs JA. Comparative study of cefuroxime axetil versus amoxicillin in children with early Lyme disease. Pediatrics. 2002 Jun;109(6):1173-7. PMID:12042561

Ergin C, Akkaya Y, Kiriş Satılmış O, Yılmaz C. [Comparison of the indirect immunofluorescence assay performance of bartonella henselae antigens obtained by co-cultivation in vero and HeLa cells].[Article in Turkish]. Mikrobiyol Bul. 2011 Jul;45(3):461-7. PMID:21935779

Eschner AK. Effect of passive immunoglobulin transfer on results of diagnostic tests for antibodies against Borrelia burgdorferi in pups born to a seropositive dam. Vet Ther. 2008 Fall;9(3):184-91. PMID:19003779

Exner MM, Lewinski MA. Isolation and detection of Borrelia burgdorferi DNA from cerebral spinal fluid, synovial fluid, blood, urine, and ticks using the Roche MagNA Pure system and real-time PCR. Diagn Microbiol Infect Dis. 2003 Aug;46(4):235-40. PMID:12944012

Feder HM Jr, Abeles M, Bernstein M, Whitaker-Worth D, Grant-Kels JM. Diagnosis, treatment, and prognosis of erythema migrans and Lyme arthritis. Clin Dermatol. 2006 Nov-Dec;24(6):509-20. PMID:17113969

Feng S, Kasten RW, Werner JA, Hodzic E, Barthold SW, Chomel BB. Immunogenicity of Bartonella henselae P26 in cats. Vet Immunol Immunopathol. 2009 Dec 15;132(2-4):251-6. Epub 2009 May 18. PMID:19500857

Fenimore A, Varanat M, Maggi R, Schultheiss P, Breitschwerdt E, Lappin MR. Bartonella spp. DNA in cardiac tissues from dogs in Colorado and Wyoming. J Vet Intern Med. 2011 May-Jun;25(3):613-6. PMID:21539606

Fonollosa A, Galdos M, Artaraz J, Perez-Irezabal J, Martinez-Alday N. Occlusive vasculitis and optic disk neovascularization associated with neuroretinitis. Ocul Immunol Inflamm. 2011 Feb;19(1):62-4. Epub 2010 Oct 31. PMID:21034304

Font RL, Del Valle M, Mitchell BM, Boniuk M. Cat-scratch uveitis confirmed by histological, serological, and molecular diagnoses. Cornea. 2011 Apr;30(4):468-71. PMID:21099401

Fournier PE, Thuny F, Richet H, Lepidi H, Casalta JP, Arzouni JP, Maurin M, Célard M, Mainardi JL, Caus T, Collart F, Habib G, Raoult D. Comprehensive diagnostic strategy for blood culture-negative endocarditis: a prospective study of 819 new cases. Clin Infect Dis. 2010 Jul 15;51(2):131-40. PMID:20540619

Gan JJ, Mandell AM, Otis JA, Holmuhamedova M, Perloff MD. Suspecting optic neuritis, diagnosing Bartonella cat scratch disease. Arch Neurol. 2011 Jan;68(1):122-6. PMID:21220684

Gardner GC, Kadel NJ. Ordering and interpreting rheumatologic laboratory tests. J Am Acad Orthop Surg. 2003 Jan-Feb;11(1):60-7. PMID:12699372

Garro AC, Rutman M, Simonsen K, Jaeger JL, Chapin K, Lockhart G. Prospective validation of a clinical prediction model for Lyme meningitis in children. Pediatrics. 2009 May;123(5):e829-34. PMID:19403476

Gaumond G, Tyropolis A, Grodzicki S, Bushmich S. Comparison of direct fluorescent antibody staining and real-time polymerase chain reaction for the detection of Borrelia burgdorferi in Ixodes scapularis ticks. J Vet Diagn Invest. 2006 Nov;18(6):583-6. PMID:17121087

Geng Z, Hou XX, Wan KL, Hao Q. [Isolation and identification of Borrelia burgdorferi sensu lato from ticks in six provinces in China]. [Article in Chinese]. Zhonghua Liu Xing Bing Xue Za Zhi. 2010 Dec;31(12):1346-1348. PMID:21223661

Girard YA, Fedorova N, Lane RS. Genetic diversity of Borrelia burgdorferi and detection of B. bissettii-like DNA in serum of north-coastal California residents. J Clin Microbiol. 2011 Mar;49(3):945-54. Epub 2010 Dec 22. PMID:21177909

Glatz M, Fingerle V, Wilske B, Ambros-Rudolph C, Kerl H, Müllegger RR. Immunoblot analysis of the seroreactivity to recombinant Borrelia burgdorferi sensu lato antigens, including VlsE, in the long-term course of treated patients with erythema migrans. Dermatology. 2008;216(2):93-103. Epub 2008 Jan 23. PMID:18216470

Glatz M, Golestani M, Kerl H, Müllegger RR. Clinical relevance of different IgG and IgM serum antibody responses to Borrelia burgdorferi after antibiotic therapy for erythema migrans: long-term follow-up study of 113 patients. Arch Dermatol. 2006 Jul;142(7):862-8. PMID:16847202

Godfroid E, Min Hu C, Humair PF, Bollen A, Gern L. PCR-reverse line blot typing method underscores the genomic heterogeneity of Borrelia valaisiana species and suggests its potential involvement in Lyme disease. J Clin Microbiol. 2003 Aug;41(8):3690-8. PMID:12904377

Goldstein RE, Cordner AP, Sandler JL, Bellohusen BA, Erb HN. Microalbuminuria and comparison of serologic testing for exposure to Borrelia burgdorferi in nonclinical Labrador and Golden Retrievers. J Vet Diagn Invest. 2007 May;19(3):294-7. PMID:17459861

Gooskens J, Templeton KE, Claas EC, van Dam AP. Evaluation of an internally controlled real-time PCR targeting the ospA gene for detection of Borrelia burgdorferi sensu lato DNA in cerebrospinal fluid. Clin Microbiol Infect. 2006 Sep;12(9):894-900. PMID:16882295

Gouriet F, Samson L, Delaage M, Mainardi JL, Meconi S, Drancourt M, Raoult D. Multiplexed whole bacterial antigen microarray, a new format for the automation of serodiagnosis: the culture-negative endocarditis paradigm. Clin Microbiol Infect. 2008 Dec;14(12):1112-8. PMID:19076842

Greco T Jr, Conti-Kelly A, Greco T. Antiphospholipid antibodies in patients with purported 'chronic Lyme disease'. Lupus. 2011;20(13):1372-7. Epub 2011 Jul 5. PMID:21729977

Grumbkow PV, Zipp A, Seidenberg V, Fehren-Schmitz L, Kempf VA, Groß U, Hummel S. Brief communication: Evidence of Bartonella quintana infections in skeletons of a historical mass grave in Kassel, Germany. Am J Phys Anthropol. 2011 Sep;146(1):134-137. PMID:21710687

Gulati A, Yalamanchili S, Golnik KC, Lee AG. Cat Scratch Neuroretinitis: The Role of Acute and Convalescent Titers for Diagnosis. J Neuroophthalmol. 2011 Sep 21. [Epub ahead of print]. PMID:21941214

Guptill L. Bartonellosis. Vet Microbiol. 2010 Jan 27;140(3-4):347-59. Epub 2009 Nov 18. PMID:20018462

Guptill L. Feline bartonellosis. Vet Clin North Am Small Anim Pract. 2010 Nov;40(6):1073-90. PMID:20933137

Haddad FA, Nadelman RB. Lyme disease and the heart. Front Biosci. 2003 Sep 1;8:s769-82. PMID:12957829

Halperin JJ. Nervous system Lyme disease. Vector Borne Zoonotic Dis. 2002 Winter;2(4):241-7. PMID:12804165

Hamer SA, Tsao JI, Walker ED, Mansfield LS, Foster ES, Hickling GJ. Use of tick surveys and serosurveys to evaluate pet dogs as a sentinel species for emerging Lyme disease. Am J Vet Res. 2009 Jan;70(1):49-56. PMID:19119948

Hassler D, Schnauffer M, Ehrfeld H, Müller E. Disappearance of specific immune response after successful therapy of chronic Lyme borreliosis. Int J Med Microbiol. 2004 Apr;293 Suppl 37:161-4. PMID:15147000

Hengge UR, Tannapfel A, Tyring SK, Erbel R, Arendt G, Ruzicka T. Lyme borreliosis. Lancet Infect Dis. 2003 Aug;3(8):489-500. PMID:12901891

Hernandez-Da-Mota S, Escalante-Razo F. Bartonellosis causing bilateral Leber neuroretinitis: a case report. Eur J Ophthalmol. 2009 Mar-Apr;19(2):307-9. PMID:19253255

Heyman P, Cochez C, Bigaignon G, Guillaume B, Zizi M, Vandenvelde C. Human Granulocytic Ehrlichiosis in Belgium: an underestimated cause of disease. J Infect. 2003 Aug;47(2):129-32. PMID:12860146

Hoey JG, Valois-Cruz F, Goldenberg H, Voskoboynik Y, Pfiffner J, Tilton RC, Mordechai E, Adelson ME. Development of an immunoglobulin M capture-based enzyme-linked immunosorbent assay for diagnosis of acute infections with Bartonella henselae. Clin Vaccine Immunol. 2009 Feb;16(2):282-4. Epub 2008 Dec 3. PMID:19052161

Holmes NE, Opat S, Kelman A, Korman TM. Refractory Bartonella quintana bacillary angiomatosis following chemotherapy for chronic lymphocytic leukaemia. J Med Microbiol. 2011 Jan;60(Pt 1):142-6. Epub 2010 Oct 14. PMID:20947664

Holmgren AR, Matteson EL. Lyme myositis. Arthritis Rheum. 2006 Aug;54(8):2697-700. PMID:16871548

Houck JA, Hojgaard A, Piesman J, Kuchta RD. Low-density microarrays for the detection of Borrelia burgdorferi s.s. (the Lyme disease spirochete) in nymphal Ixodes scapularis.   Ticks Tick Borne Dis. 2011 Mar;2(1):27-36. Epub 2010 Nov 27. PMID:21771534

Hristea A, Hristescu S, Ciufecu C, Vasile A. Seroprevalence of Borrelia burgdorferi in Romania. Eur J Epidemiol. 2001;17(9):891-6. PMID:12081110

Hsieh JW, Tung KC, Chen WC, Lin JW, Chien LJ, Hsu YM, Wang HC, Chomel BB, Chang CC. Epidemiology of Bartonella infection in rodents and shrews in Taiwan. Zoonoses Public Health. 2010 Sep;57(6):439-46. PMID:19538457

Huang J, Dai L, Lei S, Liao DY, Wang XQ, Luo TY, Chen Y, Hang ZB, Li GD, Dong DD, Xu G, Gu ZC, Hao JL, Hua P, He L, Duan FL. [Application of Warthin-Starry stain, immunohistochemistry and transmission electron microscopy in diagnosis of cat scratch disease].[Article in Chinese]. Zhonghua Bing Li Xue Za Zhi. 2010 Apr;39(4):225-9. PMID:20654119

Hufschmidt A, Müller-Felber W, Tzitiridou M, Fietzek UM, Haberl C, Heinen F. Canalicular magnetic stimulation lacks specificity to differentiate idiopathic facial palsy from borreliosis in children. Eur J Paediatr Neurol. 2008 Sep;12(5):366-70. Epub 2008 Feb 21. PMID:18206409

Hunfeld KP, Ernst M, Zachary P, Jaulhac B, Sonneborn HH, Brade V. Development and laboratory evaluation of a new recombinant ELISA for the serodiagnosis of Lyme disease. Wien Klin Wochenschr. 2002 Jul 31;114(13-14):580-5. PMID:12422605

Hunfeld KP, Kraiczy P, Kekoukh E, Schäfer V, Brade V. Standardised in vitro susceptibility testing of Borrelia burgdorferi against well-known and newly developed antimicrobial agents--possible implications for new therapeutic approaches to Lyme disease. Int J Med Microbiol. 2002 Jun;291 Suppl 33:125-37. PMID:12141737

Hunfeld KP, Ruzic-Sabljic E, Norris DE, Kraiczy P, Strle F. In vitro susceptibility testing of Borrelia burgdorferi sensu lato isolates cultured from patients with erythema migrans before and after antimicrobial chemotherapy. Antimicrob Agents Chemother. 2005 Apr;49(4):1294-301. PMID:15793100

Hunfeld KP, Stanek G, Straube E, Hagedorn HJ, Schörner C, Mühlschlegel F, Brade V. Quality of Lyme disease serology. Lessons from the German Proficiency Testing Program 1999-2001. A preliminary report. Wien Klin Wochenschr. 2002 Jul 31;114(13-14):591-600. PMID:12422607

Hunt PW. Molecular diagnosis of infections and resistance in veterinary and human parasites. Vet Parasitol. 2011 Aug 4;180(1-2):12-46. Epub 2011 May 27. PMID:21700392

Irshad FA, Gordon RA. Bartonella henselae neuroretinitis in a 15-year-old girl with chronic myelogenous leukemia. J AAPOS. 2009 Dec;13(6):602-4. PMID:20006827

Ivacic L, Reed KD, Mitchell PD, Ghebranious N. A LightCycler TaqMan assay for detection of Borrelia burgdorferi sensu lato in clinical samples. Diagn Microbiol Infect Dis. 2007 Feb;57(2):137-43. Epub 2006 Sep 20. PMID:16989975

Jacobs DJ, Scott ML, Slusher MM. Localised retinal vasculitis in cat scratch disease. BMJ Case Rep. 2009;2009. pii: bcr09.2008.0904. Epub 2009 Mar 17. PMID:21686569

Jäderlund KH, Egenvall A, Bergström K, Hedhammar A. Seroprevalence of Borrelia burgdorferi sensu lato and Anaplasma phagocytophilum in dogs with neurological signs. Vet Rec. 2007 Jun 16;160(24):825-31. PMID:17575245

James FM, Engiles JB, Beech J. Meningitis, cranial neuritis, and radiculoneuritis associated with Borrelia burgdorferi infection in a horse. J Am Vet Med Assoc. 2010 Nov 15;237(10):1180-5. PMID:21073390

Jeanclaude D, Godmer P, Leveiller D, Pouedras P, Fournier PE, Raoult D, Rolain JM. Bartonella alsatica endocarditis in a French patient in close contact with rabbits. Clin Microbiol Infect. 2009 Dec;15 Suppl 2:110-1. Epub 2009 Apr 30. PMID:19438633

Jennings F, Lambert E, Fredericson M. Rheumatic diseases presenting as sports-related injuries. Sports Med. 2008;38(11):917-30. PMID:18937522

Jobe DA, Lovrich SD, Asp KE, Mathiason MA, Albrecht SE, Schell RF, Callister SM. Significantly improved accuracy of diagnosis of early Lyme disease by peptide enzyme-linked immunosorbent assay based on the borreliacidal antibody epitope of Borrelia burgdorferi OspC. Clin Vaccine Immunol. 2008 Jun;15(6):981-5. Epub 2008 Apr 16. PMID:18329555

Johnson JL, Ginsberg HS, Zhioua E, Whitworth UG Jr, Markowski D, Hyland KE, Hu R. Passive tick surveillance, dog seropositivity, and incidence of human lyme disease. Vector Borne Zoonotic Dis. 2004 Summer;4(2):137-42. PMID:15228814

Johnson L, Aylward A, Stricker RB. Healthcare access and burden of care for patients with Lyme disease: a large United States survey. Health Policy. 2011 Sep;102(1):64-71. Epub 2011 Jun 14. PMID:21676482

Johnson L, Stricker RB. Treatment of Lyme disease: a medicolegal assessment. Expert Rev Anti Infect Ther. 2004 Aug;2(4):533-57. PMID:15482219

Juchnowicz D, Rudnik I, Czernikiewicz A, Zajkowska J, Pancewicz SA. [Mental disorders in the course of lyme borreliosis and tick borne encephalitis].[Article in Polish]. Przegl Epidemiol. 2002;56 Suppl 1:37-50. PMID:12194228

Kaçar N, Taşli L, Demirkan N, Ergin C, Ergin S. HIV-negative case of bacillary angiomatosis with chronic hepatitis B. J Dermatol. 2010 Aug;37(8):722-5. PMID:20649715

Kaiser PO, Riess T, O'Rourke F, Linke D, Kempf VA. Bartonella spp.: throwing light on uncommon human infections. Int J Med Microbiol. 2011 Jan;301(1):7-15. Epub 2010 Sep 15. PMID:20833105

Kalogeropoulos C, Koumpoulis I, Mentis A, Pappa C, Zafeiropoulos P, Aspiotis M. Bartonella and intraocular inflammation: a series of cases and review of literature. Clin Ophthalmol. 2011;5:817-29. Epub 2011 Jun 16. PMID:21750616

Kamoi K, Yoshida T, Takase H, Yokota M, Kawaguchi T, Mochizuki M. Seroprevalence of Bartonella henselae in patients with uveitis and healthy individuals in Tokyo. Jpn J Ophthalmol. 2009 Sep;53(5):490-3. Epub 2009 Oct 22. PMID:19847604

Kanjwal K, Karabin B, Kanjwal Y, Grubb BP. Postural orthostatic tachycardia syndrome following Lyme disease. Cardiol J. 2011;18(1):63-6. PMID:21305487

Kantas I, Katotomichelakis M, Vafiadis M, Kaloutsa ZV, Papadakis CE. Serous labyrinthitis as a manifestation of cat scratch disease: a case report. J Med Case Reports. 2009 Sep 15;3:7405. PMID:20519021

Karan' LS, Koliasnikova NM, Toporkova MG, Makhneva MA, Nadezhdina MV, Esaulkova AIu, Romanenko VV, Arumova EA, Platonov AE, Maleev VV. [Usage of real time polymerase chain reaction for diagnostics of different tick-borne infections].[Article in Russian]. Zh Mikrobiol Epidemiol Immunobiol. 2010 May-Jun;(3):72-7. PMID:20734723

Karolak J, Gotz-Wipckowska A. [Neuroretinitis in cat scratch disease]. [Article in Polish]. Klin Oczna. 2010;112(4-6):131-4. PMID:20825068

Karosi T, Rácz T, Szekanecz E, Tóth A, Sziklai I. Recurrent laryngeal nerve paralysis due to subclinical Lyme borreliosis. J Laryngol Otol. 2010 Mar;124(3):336-8. Epub 2009 Sep 10. PMID:19740453

Karris MY, Litwin CM, Dong HS, Vinetz J. Bartonella henselae Infection of Prosthetic Aortic Valve Associated with Colitis. Vector Borne Zoonotic Dis. 2011 Nov;11(11):1503-5. Epub 2011 Jun 24. PMID:21702667

Kaufmann J, Buccola JM, Stead W, Rowley C, Wong M, Bates CK. Secondary symptomatic parvovirus B19 infection in a healthy adult. J Gen Intern Med. 2007 Jun;22(6):877-8. Epub 2007 Mar 24. PMID:17384979

Kaya AD, Parlak AH, Ozturk CE, Behcet M. Seroprevalence of Borrelia burgdorferi infection among forestry workers and farmers in Duzce, north-western Turkey. New Microbiol. 2008 Apr;31(2):203-9. PMID:18623985

Kelly JJ. Evaluation of peripheral neuropathy. Part III: vasculitic, infectious, inherited, and idiopathic neuropathies. Rev Neurol Dis. 2005 Spring;2(2):70-9. PMID:19813300

Khoudri I, Frémont G, Flageul B, Brière J, Dubertret L, Viguier M. [Bilateral inguinal lymphadenopathy and erythema nodosum: an uncommon presentation of cat scratch disease].[Article in French]. Rev Med Interne. 2011 Mar;32(3):e34-6. Epub 2010 Jun 19. PMID:20646798

Kim D, Kordick D, Divers T, Chang YF. In vitro susceptibilities of Leptospira spp. and Borrelia burgdorferi isolates to amoxicillin, tilmicosin, and enrofloxacin. J Vet Sci. 2006 Dec;7(4):355-9. PMID:17106227

Klotz SA, Ianas V, Elliott SP. Cat-scratch Disease. Am Fam Physician. 2011 Jan 15;83(2):152-5. PMID:21243990

Koga T, Taguchi J, Suzuki M, Higa Y, Kamimura T, Nishimura M, Arakawa M. Cat scratch disease presenting with a retroperitoneal abscess in a patient without animal contacts. J Infect Chemother. 2009 Dec;15(6):414-6. PMID:20012734

Koneva OA, Anan'eva LP, Shtannikov AV, Evsegneev SI, Baranova EV. [Comparative analysis of use of two strains of various genotypes of Borrelia burgdorferi sensu lato as antigens for antibody identification in Ixodes tick borreliosis by indirect immunofluorescence].[Article in Russian]. Klin Lab Diagn. 2003 May;(5):41-3. PMID:12822309

Koo M, Manalili S, Bankowski MJ, Sampath R, Hofstadler SA, Koo J. A "silent culture-negative" abdominal aortic mycotic aneurysm: Rapid detection of Bartonella species using PCR and high-throughput mass spectrometry. Hawaii Med J. 2010 Mar;69(3):68-9. PMID:20397506

Kornreich BG, Craven M, McDonough SP, Nydam DV, Scorza V, Assarasakorn S, Lappin M, Simpson KW. Fluorescence In-situ Hybridization for the Identification of Bacterial Species in Archival Heart Valve Sections of Canine Bacterial Endocarditis. J Comp Pathol. 2011 Oct 24. [Epub ahead of print]. PMID:22030263

Krause PJ, McKay K, Thompson CA, Sikand VK, Lentz R, Lepore T, Closter L, Christianson D, Telford SR, Persing D, Radolf JD, Spielman A; Deer-Associated Infection Study Group. Disease-specific diagnosis of coinfecting tickborne zoonoses: babesiosis, human granulocytic ehrlichiosis, and Lyme disease. Clin Infect Dis. 2002 May 1;34(9):1184-91. Epub 2002 Apr 4. PMID:11941544

Krupka I, Knauer J, Lorentzen L, O'Connor TP, Saucier J, Straubinger RK. Borrelia burgdorferi sensu lato species in Europe induce diverse immune responses against C6 peptides in infected mice. Clin Vaccine Immunol. 2009 Nov;16(11):1546-62. Epub 2009 Sep 2. PMID:19726618

Krupka I, Straubinger RK. Lyme borreliosis in dogs and cats: background, diagnosis, treatment and prevention of infections with Borrelia burgdorferi sensu stricto. Vet Clin North Am Small Anim Pract. 2010 Nov;40(6):1103-19. PMID:20933139

Kubicka-Trzaska A, Oleksy P, Karska-Basta I, Romanowska-Dixon
B. [Acute posterior multifocal placoid pigment epitheliopathy
(APMPPE)—a therapeutic dilemma].[Article in Polish]. Klin Oczna.
2010;112(4-6):127-30. PMID:20825067

Kubová Z, Szanyi J, Langrová J, Kremlácek J, Kuba M, Honegr
K. Motion-onset and pattern-reversal visual evoked potentials
in diagnostics of neuroborreliosis. J Clin Neurophysiol. 2006
Oct;23(5):416-20. PMID:17016151

Kvasnicka HM, Thiele J. [Differentiation of granulomatous
lesions in the bone marrow].[Article in German]. Pathologe. 2002
Nov;23(6):465-71. Epub 2002 Oct 8. PMID:12436300

Lagal V, Postic D, Ruzic-Sabljic E, Baranton G. Genetic diversity
among Borrelia strains determined by single-strand conformation
polymorphism analysis of the ospC gene and its association
with invasiveness. J Clin Microbiol. 2003 Nov;41(11):5059-65.
PMID:14605139

Lakos A, Reiczigel J, Solymosi N. The positive predictive value of
Borrelia burgdorferi serology in the light of symptoms of patients sent
to an outpatient service for tick-borne diseases. Inflamm Res. 2010
Nov;59(11):959-64. Epub 2010 May 13. PMID:20461540

Lange D, Oeder C, Waltermann K, Mueller A, Oehme A, Rohrberg
R, Marsch W, Fischer M. Bacillary angiomatosis. [Article in
English, German]. J Dtsch Dermatol Ges. 2009 Sep;7(9):767-69.
PMID:19298547

Ledue TB, Collins MF, Young J, Schriefer ME. Evaluation of the
recombinant VlsE-based liaison chemiluminescence immunoassay for
detection of Borrelia burgdorferi and diagnosis of Lyme disease. Clin
Vaccine Immunol. 2008 Dec;15(12):1796-804. Epub 2008 Oct 22.
PMID:18945880

Lemos ER, Mares-Guia MA, Almeida DN, Silva RG, Silva CM, Britto C, Lamas CC. [Traveler's fever associated with cervical adenomegaly and antibodies for Bartonella sp in a Brazilian patient returning from South Africa].[Article in Portuguese]. Rev Soc Bras Med Trop. 2010 Jul-Aug;43(4):472-3. PMID:20802956

Lencáková D, Fingerle V, Stefancíková A, Schulte-Spechtel U, Petko B, Schréter I, Wilske B. Evaluation of recombinant line immunoblot for detection of Lyme disease in Slovakia: comparison with two other immunoassays. Vector Borne Zoonotic Dis. 2008 Jun;8(3):381-90. PMID:18279004

Lesseva M, Christova I, Miloshev G. Cloning and expression of recombinant flagellar protein flaB from Borrelia burgdorferi. Folia Med (Plovdiv). 2007;49(3-4):58-62. PMID:18504936

Levy S, O'Connor TP, Hanscom JL, Shields P. Utility of an in-office C6 ELISA test kit for determination of infection status of dogs naturally exposed to Borrelia burgdorferi. Vet Ther. 2002 Fall;3(3):308-15. PMID:12447839

Lienhardt B, Irani S, Gaspert A, Weishaupt D, Boehler A. Disseminated infection with Bartonella henselae in a lung transplant recipient. J Heart Lung Transplant. 2009 Jul;28(7):736-9. PMID:19560704

Lin EY, Tsigrelis C, Baddour LM, Lepidi H, Rolain JM, Patel R, Raoult D. Candidatus Bartonella mayotimonensis and endocarditis. Emerg Infect Dis. 2010 Mar;16(3):500-3. PMID:20202430

Littman MP. Canine borreliosis. Vet Clin North Am Small Anim Pract. 2003 Jul;33(4):827-62. PMID:12910746

Ljøstad U, Skarpaas T, Mygland A. Clinical usefulness of intrathecal antibody testing in acute Lyme neuroborreliosis. Eur J Neurol. 2007 Aug;14(8):873-6. PMID:17662007

Loeckx I, Tuerlinckx D, Jespers S, Marchant AS, Bodart E. [A clinical case of spontaneous involution of systemic cat scratch disease].[Article in French]. Rev Med Liege. 2010 Feb;65(2):78-80. PMID:20344917

López-Alberola RF. Neuroborreliosis and the pediatric population: a review. Rev Neurol. 2006 Apr 10;42 Suppl 3:S91-6. PMID:16642458

Lünemann JD, Gelderblom H, Sospedra M, Quandt JA, Pinilla C, Marques A, Martin R. Cerebrospinal fluid-infiltrating CD4+ T cells recognize Borrelia burgdorferi lysine-enriched protein domains and central nervous system autoantigens in early lyme encephalitis. Infect Immun. 2007 Jan;75(1):243-51. Epub 2006 Oct 23. PMID:17060473

Lynch T, Iverson J, Kosoy M. Combining culture techniques for Bartonella: the best of both worlds. J Clin Microbiol. 2011 Apr;49(4):1363-8. Epub 2011 Feb 2. PMID:21289156

Macarez R, Bazin S, Lagauche D, Soullié B, Giordano P, May F, Guigon B. [Onset of Leber's hereditary optic neuropathy in association with borreliosis].[Article in French]. J Fr Ophtalmol. 2005 Dec;28(10):1095-100. PMID:16395203

Macdonald K. Infective endocarditis in dogs: diagnosis and therapy. Vet Clin North Am Small Anim Pract. 2010 Jul;40(4):665-84. PMID:20610018

Magalhães RF, Cintra ML, Barjas-Castro ML, Del Negro GM, Okay TS, Velho PE. Blood donor infected with Bartonella henselae. Transfus Med. 2010 Aug 1;20(4):280-2. Epub 2010 Mar 24. PMID:20345384

Magalhães RF, Urso Pitassi LH, Lania BG, Barjas-Castro ML, Neves Ferreira Velho PE. Bartonellosis as cause of death after red blood cell unit transfusion. Ultrastruct Pathol. 2009 Jul-Aug;33(4):151-4. PMID:19728230

Maggi RG, Mascarelli PE, Pultorak EL, Hegarty BC, Bradley JM, Mozayeni BR, Breitschwerdt EB. Bartonella spp. bacteremia in high-risk immunocompetent patients. Diagn Microbiol Infect Dis. 2011 Dec;71(4):430-7. Epub 2011 Oct 13. PMID:21996096

Maggi RG, Reichelt S, Toliver M, Engber B. Borrelia species in Ixodes affinis and Ixodes scapularis ticks collected from the coastal plain of North Carolina. Ticks Tick Borne Dis. 2010 Dec;1(4):168-71. Epub 2010 Oct 20. PMID:21771524

Magnarelli LA, Bushmich SL, IJdo JW, Fikrig E. Seroprevalence of antibodies against Borrelia burgdorferi and Anaplasma phagocytophilum in cats. Am J Vet Res. 2005 Nov;66(11):1895-9. PMID:16334946

Magnarelli LA, Lawrenz M, Norris SJ, Fikrig E. Comparative reactivity of human sera to recombinant VlsE and other Borrelia burgdorferi antigens in class-specific enzyme-linked immunosorbent assays for Lyme borreliosis. J Med Microbiol. 2002 Aug;51(8):649-55. PMID:12171295

Magnarelli LA, Stafford KC 3rd, Ijdo JW, Fikrig E. Antibodies to whole-cell or recombinant antigens of Borrelia burgdorferi, Anaplasma phagocytophilum, and Babesia microti in white-footed mice. J Wildl Dis. 2006 Oct;42(4):732-8. PMID:17255439

Magri JM, Johnson MT, Herring TA, Greenblatt JF. Lyme disease knowledge, beliefs, and practices of New Hampshire primary care physicians. J Am Board Fam Pract. 2002 Jul-Aug;15(4):277-84. PMID:12150460

Maguiña C, Guerra H, Ventosilla P. Bartonellosis. Clin Dermatol. 2009 May-Jun;27(3):271-80. PMID:19362689

Manalai P, Bhalavat RM, Dobbs MR, Lippmann S. Coma falsely attributed to Lyme disease. J Ky Med Assoc. 2008 Jul;106(7):317-9. PMID:18777697

Marangoni A, Moroni A, Accardo S, Cevenini R. Borrelia burgdorferi VlsE antigen for the serological diagnosis of Lyme borreliosis. Eur J Clin Microbiol Infect Dis. 2008 May;27(5):349-54. Epub 2008 Jan 16. PMID:18197445

Marienfeld CB, Dicapua DB, Sze GK, Goldstein JM. Expressive aphasia as a presentation of encephalitis with Bartonella henselae infection in an immunocompetent adult. Yale J Biol Med. 2010 Jun;83(2):67-71. PMID:20589186

Martín L, Vidal L, Campins A, Salvá F, Riera M, Carrillo A, Sáez de Ibarra JI. Bartonella as a cause of blood culture-negative endocarditis. Description of five cases. [Article in English, Spanish]. Rev Esp Cardiol. 2009 Jun;62(6):694-7. PMID:19480767

Martinez-Diaz GJ, Kim J, Bruckner AL. A toddler with facial nodules: a case of idiopathic facial aseptic granuloma. Dermatol Online J. 2010 Jan 15;16(1):9. PMID:20137751

Marques AR, Hornung RL, Dally L, Philipp MT. Detection of immune complexes is not independent of detection of antibodies in Lyme disease patients and does not confirm active infection with Borrelia burgdorferi. Clin Diagn Lab Immunol. 2005 Sep;12(9):1036-40. PMID:16148168

Maruyama S. [Cat-scratch disease].[Article in Japanese]. Nihon Rinsho. 2010 Jun;68 Suppl 6:244-7. PMID:20942049

Mastrandrea S, Simonetta Taras M, Capitta P, Tola S, Marras V, Strusi G, Masala G. Detection of Bartonella henselae--DNA in macronodular hepatic lesions of an immunocompetent woman. Clin Microbiol Infect. 2009 Dec;15 Suppl 2:116-7. Epub 2009 Sep 28. PMID:19793123

Mavin S, Evans R, Milner RM, Chatterton JM, Ho-Yen DO. Local Borrelia burgdorferi sensu stricto and Borrelia afzelii strains in a single mixed antigen improves western blot sensitivity. J Clin Pathol. 2009 Jun;62(6):552-4. Epub 2009 Feb 23. PMID:19240047

Mavin S, Hopkins PC, MacLennan A, Joss AW, Ho-Yen DO. Urban and rural risks of Lyme disease in the Scottish Highlands. Scott Med J. 2009 May;54(2):24-6. PMID:19530498

Mavin S, McDonagh S, Evans R, Milner RM, Chatterton JM, Ho-Yen DO. Interpretation criteria in Western blot diagnosis of Lyme borreliosis. Br J Biomed Sci. 2011;68(1):5-10. PMID:21473255

Mazepa AW, Kidd LB, Young KM, Trepanier LA. Clinical presentation of 26 anaplasma phagocytophilum-seropositive dogs residing in an endemic area. J Am Anim Hosp Assoc. 2010 Nov-Dec;46(6):405-12. PMID:21041333

McGinnis J, Bohnker BK, Malakooti M, Mann M, Sack DM. Lyme disease reporting for Navy and Marine Corps (1997-2000). Mil Med. 2003 Dec;168(12):1011-4. PMID:14719627

Mead P. Lyme disease testing. Lancet Infect Dis. 2006 Mar;6(3):122-3. PMID:16500589

Metz CH, Buer J, Bornfeld N, Lipski A. Bilateral Bartonella henselae neuroretinitis with stellate maculopathy in a 6-year-old boy. Infection. 2011 Aug 9. [Epub ahead of print]. PMID:21826435

Meyniel C, Wiertlewski S. [Optic neuritis].[Article in French]. Rev Med Interne. 2010 Jul;31(7):481-5. PMID:20434241

Michos A, Dessypris N, Pourtsidis A, Moschovi M, Polychronopoulou S, Athanasiadou-Piperopoulou F, Kalmanti M, Syriopoulou VP, Mavrouli MD, Petridou ET. Delayed exposure to infections and childhood lymphomas: a case-control study. Cancer Causes Control. 2009 Jul;20(5):795-802. Epub 2009 Jan 25. PMID:19169895

Mietze A, Morick D, Köhler H, Harrus S, Dehio C, Nolte I, Goethe R. Combined MLST and AFLP typing of Bartonella henselae isolated from cats reveals new sequence types and suggests clonal evolution. Vet Microbiol. 2011 Mar 24;148(2-4):238-45. Epub 2010 Sep 21. PMID:20863631

Misić-Majerus L, Bujić N. Madarić V, Avsic-Zupanc T. [An abortive type of tick-borne meningoencephalitis].[Article in Croatian]. Acta Med Croatica. 2003;57(2):111-6. PMID:12879690

Mitchell BM, Font RL. Molecular detection of Bartonella henselae for the diagnosis of cat scratch disease and bacillary angiomatosis of the conjunctiva. Cornea. 2011 Jul;30(7):807-14. PMID:21282991

Mofenson LM, Brady MT, Danner SP, Dominguez KL, Hazra R, Handelsman E, Havens P, Nesheim S, Read JS, Serchuck L, Van Dyke R; Centers for Disease Control and Prevention; National Institutes of Health; HIV Medicine Association of the Infectious Diseases Society of America; Pediatric Infectious Diseases Society; American Academy of Pediatrics. Guidelines for the Prevention and Treatment of Opportunistic Infections among HIV-exposed and HIV-infected children: recommendations from CDC, the National Institutes of Health, the HIV Medicine Association of the Infectious Diseases Society of America, the Pediatric Infectious Diseases Society, and the American Academy of Pediatrics. MMWR Recomm Rep. 2009 Sep 4;58(RR-11):1-166. PMID:19730409

Montcriol A, Benard F, Fenollar F, Ribeiri A, Bonnet M, Collart F, Guidon C. Fatal myocarditis-associated Bartonella quintana endocarditis: a case report. J Med Case Reports. 2009 Jul 17;3:7325. PMID:19830188

Morrison C, Seifter A, Aucott JN. Unusual presentation of Lyme disease: Horner syndrome with negative serology. J Am Board Fam Med. 2009 Mar-Apr;22(2):219-22. PMID:19264948

Morway C, Kosoy M, Eisen R, Montenieri J, Sheff K, Reynolds PJ, Powers N. A longitudinal study of Bartonella infection in populations of woodrats and their fleas. J Vector Ecol. 2008 Dec;33(2):353-64. PMID:19263856

Mrázek V, Bartůněk P, Varejka P, Janovská D, Bína R, Hulínská D. [Prevalence of antiborrelia antibodies in two populations: various interpretations of the same data].[Article in Czech]. Epidemiol Mikrobiol Imunol. 2002 Feb;51(1):19-22. PMID:11881295

Muenzel D, Duetsch S, Fauser C, Slotta-Huspenina J, Gaa J, Rummeny EJ, Holzapfel K. Diffusion-weighted magnetic resonance imaging in cervical lymphadenopathy: report of three cases of patients with Bartonella henselae infection mimicking malignant disease. Acta Radiol. 2009 Oct;50(8):914-6. PMID:19636985

Mullegger RR, Glatz M. Is serological follow-up useful for patients with cutaneous Lyme borreliosis? Curr Probl Dermatol. 2009;37:178-82. Epub 2009 Apr 8. PMID:19367102

Müller NF, Kaiser PO, Linke D, Schwarz H, Riess T, Schäfer A, Eble JA, Kempf VA. Trimeric autotransporter adhesin-dependent adherence of Bartonella henselae, Bartonella quintana, and Yersinia enterocolitica to matrix components and endothelial cells under static and dynamic flow conditions. Infect Immun. 2011 Jul;79(7):2544-53. Epub 2011 May 2. PMID:21536788

Murdoch W, Rosin FC. One presentation, two continents: left wrist myositis of distinct etiology in genetically similar individuals. J Am Board Fam Med. 2009 Jul-Aug;22(4):408-11. PMID:19587255

Murray MA, Zamecki KJ, Paskowski J, Lelli GJ Jr. Ocular bacillary angiomatosis in an immunocompromised man. Ophthal Plast Reconstr Surg. 2010 Sep-Oct;26(5):371-2. PMID:20683276

Murray TS, Shapiro ED. Lyme disease. Clin Lab Med. 2010 Mar;30(1):311-28. PMID:20513553

Myint KS, Gibbons RV, Iverson J, Shrestha SK, Pavlin JA, Mongkolsirichaikul D, Kosoy MY. Serological response to Bartonella species in febrile patients from Nepal. Trans R Soc Trop Med Hyg. 2011 Dec;105(12):740-2. Epub 2011 Sep 28. PMID:21955739

Naesens R, Vermeiren S, Van Schaeren J, Jeurissen A. False positive Lyme serology due to syphilis: report of 6 cases and review of the literature. Acta Clin Belg. 2011 Jan-Feb;66(1):58-9. PMID:21485767

Namekata MS, Clifford DL, Kasten RW, Henn JB, Garcelon DK, Coonan TJ, Chomel BB. Seroprevalence of Bartonella spp. in the endangered island fox (Urocyon littoralis). Vet Microbiol. 2009 Apr 14;136(1-2):184-7. Epub 2008 Oct 28. PMID:19058928

Nghiem PP, Schatzberg SJ. Conventional and molecular diagnostic testing for the acute neurologic patient. J Vet Emerg Crit Care (San Antonio). 2010 Feb;20(1):46-61. PMID:20230434

Nigrovic LE, Thompson AD, Fine AM, Kimia A. Clinical predictors of Lyme disease among children with a peripheral facial palsy at an emergency department in a Lyme disease-endemic area. Pediatrics. 2008 Nov;122(5):e1080-5. Epub 2008 Oct 17. PMID:18931349

Nijssen E, Cescau S, Vayssier-Taussat M, Wang J, Biville F. Identification of mechanisms involved in iron and haem uptake in Bartonella birtlesii: in silico and in vivo approaches. Clin Microbiol Infect. 2009 Dec;15 Suppl 2:118-9. Epub 2009 Apr 30. PMID:19438629

Nishio N, Kubota T, Nakao Y, Hidaka H. Cat scratch disease with encephalopathy in a 9-year-old girl. Pediatr Int. 2008 Dec;50(6):823-4. PMID:19067901

Nunes Rosado FG, Stratton CW, Mosse CA. Clinicopathologic correlation of epidemiologic and histopathologic features of pediatric bacterial lymphadenitis. Arch Pathol Lab Med. 2011 Nov;135(11):1490-3. PMID:22032579

Occorsio P, Orso G, di Martino L. [Ticks and the pediatrician].[Article in Italian]. Parassitologia. 2004 Jun;46(1-2):115-8. PMID:15305698

O'Connor TP, Esty KJ, Hanscom JL, Shields P, Philipp MT. Dogs vaccinated with common Lyme disease vaccines do not respond to IR6, the conserved immunodominant region of the VlsE surface protein of Borrelia burgdorferi. Clin Diagn Lab Immunol. 2004 May;11(3):458-62. PMID:15138170

Oliver J, Means RG, Kogut S, Prusinski M, Howard JJ, Layne LJ, Chu FK, Reddy A, Lee L, White DJ. Prevalence of Borrelia burgdorferi in small mammals in New York state. J Med Entomol. 2006 Sep;43(5):924-35. PMID:17017230

Owen DC. Is Gulf War Syndrome actually chronic Lyme disease? Med Hypotheses. 2005;64(4):717-20. PMID:15694687

Pachner AR, Dail D, Li L, Gurey L, Feng S, Hodzic E, Barthold S. Humoral immune response associated with lyme borreliosis in nonhuman primates: analysis by immunoblotting and enzyme-linked immunosorbent assay with sonicates or recombinant proteins. Clin Diagn Lab Immunol. 2002 Nov;9(6):1348-55. PMID:12414773

Palecek T, Kuchynka P, Hulinska D, Schramlova J, Hrbackova H, Vitkova I, Simek S, Horak J, Louch WE, Linhart A. Presence of Borrelia burgdorferi in endomyocardial biopsies in patients with new-onset unexplained dilated cardiomyopathy. Med Microbiol Immunol. 2010 May;199(2):139-43. Epub 2010 Jan 6. PMID:20052487

Panic G, Stanulovic V, Popov T. Atrio-ventricular block as the first presentation of disseminated Lyme disease. Int J Cardiol. 2011 Aug 4;150(3):e104-6. Epub 2010 Mar 11. PMID:20226549

Papadopouli E, Michailidi E, Papadopoulou E, Paspalaki P, Vlahakis I, Kalmanti M. Cervical lymphadenopathy in childhood epidemiology and management. Pediatr Hematol Oncol. 2009 Sep;26(6):454-60. PMID:19657996

Pape M, Mandraveli K, Alexiou-Daniel S. Clinical aspects of Bartonella infection in northern Greece. Clin Microbiol Infect. 2009 Dec;15 Suppl 2:91-2. Epub 2009 May 18. PMID:19456804

Patil N, Bariola JR, Saccente M, Vyas KS, Bradsher RW Jr. A clinical review of Lyme disease in Arkansas. J Ark Med Soc. 2010 Feb;106(8):186-8. PMID:20218039

Pennisi MG, La Camera E, Giacobbe L, Orlandella BM, Lentini V, Zummo S, Fera MT. Molecular detection of Bartonella henselae and Bartonella clarridgeiae in clinical samples of pet cats from Southern Italy. Res Vet Sci. 2010 Jun;88(3):379-84. Epub 2009 Dec 5. PMID:19963231

Perez C, Hummel JB, Keene BW, Maggi RG, Diniz PP, Breitschwerdt EB. Successful treatment of Bartonella henselae endocarditis in a cat. J Feline Med Surg. 2010 Jun;12(6):483-6. Epub 2010 Feb 6. PMID:20138559

Pérez C, Maggi RG, Diniz PP, Breitschwerdt EB. Molecular and serological diagnosis of Bartonella infection in 61 dogs from the United States. J Vet Intern Med. 2011 Jul-Aug;25(4):805-10. Epub 2011 May 25. PMID:21615498

Pérez GJ, Munita SJ, Araos BR, López GJ, Stevenson AR, González AP, Pérez CD, Noriega RL. [Cat scratch disease associated neuroretinitis: clinical report and review of the literature].[Article in Spanish]. Rev Chilena Infectol. 2010 Oct;27(5):417-22. PMID:21186508

Peters GB 3rd, Bakri SJ, Krohel GB. Cause and prognosis of nontraumatic sixth nerve palsies in young adults. Ophthalmology. 2002 Oct;109(10):1925-8. PMID:12359616

Pfrommer S, Maier M, Mayer C, Erben A, Engelmann V, Lohmann CP. [Vasoproliferative retinal tumours].[Article in German]. Ophthalmologe. 2011 Mar;108(3):265-8. PMID:21153829

Phillips SE, Burrascano JJ, Horowitz R, Savely VR, Stricker RB. Lyme disease testing. Lancet Infect Dis. 2006 Mar;6(3):122. PMID:16500590

Piérard-Franchimont C, Quatresooz P, Piérard GE. Skin diseases associated with Bartonella infection: facts and controversies. Clin Dermatol. 2010 Sep-Oct;28(5):483-8. PMID:20797506

Pinna A, Puglia E, Dore S. Unusual retinal manifestations of cat scratch disease. Int Ophthalmol. 2011 Apr;31(2):125-8. Epub 2011 Jan 26. PMID:21267628

Pitassi LH, Cintra ML, Ferreira MR, Magalhães RF, Velho PE. Blood cell findings resembling Bartonella spp. Ultrastruct Pathol. 2010 Feb;34(1):2-6. PMID:20070147

Podsiadły E, Sapiejka E, Dabrowska-Bień J, Majkowski J, Tylewska-Wierzbanowska S. [Diagnostics of cat scratch disease and present methods of bartonellosis recognition--a case report].[Article in Polish]. Pol Merkur Lekarski. 2009 Feb;26(152):131-5. PMID:19388519

Polat E, Turhan V, Aslan M, Müsellim B, Onem Y, Ertuğrul B. [First report of three culture confirmed human Lyme cases in Turkey]. [Article in Turkish]. Mikrobiyol Bul. 2010 Jan;44(1):133-9. PMID:20455410

Pomelova VG, Kharitonenkov IG, Sadykbekova RK, Bychenkova TA, Anan'eva LP, Sokolova MV, Osin NS. [Designing and clinical testing of immune-enzyme and immunofluorescence test systems for serodiagnosis of ixodes borreliosis].[Article in Russian]. Vestn Ross Akad Med Nauk. 2004;(1):3-7. PMID:15022545

Pourel J. [Clinical diagnosis of Lyme borreliosis in case of joint and muscular presentations].[Article in French]. Med Mal Infect. 2007 Jul-Aug;37(7-8):523-31. Epub 2007 Mar 26. PMID:17368783

Probert W, Louie JK, Tucker JR, Longoria R, Hogue R, Moler S, Graves M, Palmer HJ, Cassady J, Fritz CL. Meningitis due to a "Bartonella washoensis"-like human pathogen. J Clin Microbiol. 2009 Jul;47(7):2332-5. Epub 2009 May 13. PMID:19439538

Przytuła L, Gińdzieńska-Sieśkiewicz E, Sierakowski S. [Diagnosis and treatment of Lyme arthritis].[Article in Polish]. Przegl Epidemiol. 2006;60 Suppl 1:125-30. PMID:16909789

Pulliainen AT, Dehio C. Bartonella henselae: subversion of vascular endothelial cell functions by translocated bacterial effector proteins. Int J Biochem Cell Biol. 2009 Mar;41(3):507-10. Epub 2008 Oct 25. PMID:18992392

Que YA, Moreillon P. Infective endocarditis. Nat Rev Cardiol. 2011 Jun;8(6):322-36. Epub 2011 Apr 12. PMID:21487430

Quebatte M, Dehio M, Tropel D, Basler A, Toller I, Raddatz G, Engel P, Huser S, Schein H, Lindroos HL, Andersson SG, Dehio C. The BatR/BatS two-component regulatory system controls the adaptive response of Bartonella henselae during human endothelial cell infection. J Bacteriol. 2010 Jul;192(13):3352-67. Epub 2010 Apr 23. PMID:20418395

Qureshi M, Bedlack RS, Cudkowicz ME. Lyme disease serology in amyotrophic lateral sclerosis. Muscle Nerve. 2009 Oct;40(4):626-8. PMID:19697382

Ramsey AH, Belongia EA, Chyou PH, Davis JP. Appropriateness of Lyme disease serologic testing. Ann Fam Med. 2004 Jul-Aug;2(4):341-4. PMID:15335133

Reis C, Cote M, Le Rhun D, Lecuelle B, Levin ML, Vayssier-Taussat M, Bonnet SI. Vector competence of the tick Ixodes ricinus for transmission of Bartonella birtlesii. PLoS Negl Trop Dis. 2011;5(5):e1186. Epub 2011 May 31. PMID:21655306

Reis C, Cote M, Paul RE, Bonnet S. Questing ticks in suburban forest are infected by at least six tick-borne pathogens. Vector Borne Zoonotic Dis. 2011 Jul;11(7):907-16. Epub 2010 Dec 15. PMID:21158500

Renou F, Raffray L, Gerber A, Moiton MP, Ferrandiz D, Yvin JL. [Hepatic localization of cat scratch disease in an immunocompetent patient].[Article in French]. Med Mal Infect. 2010 Mar;40(3):172-4. Epub 2009 Jul 17. PMID:19616394

Ricart JJ. [Infective endocarditis due to Bartonella quintana].[Article in Spanish]. Medicina (B Aires). 2008;68(6):478. PMID:19147434

Roberts DM, Caimano M, McDowell J, Theisen M, Holm A, Orff E, Nelson D, Wikel S, Radolf J, Marconi RT. Environmental regulation and differential production of members of the Bdr protein family of Borrelia burgdorferi. Infect Immun. 2002 Dec;70(12):7033-41. PMID:12438383

Rodríguez C M, Giachetto L G, Cuneo E A, Gutiérrez B Mdel C, Shimchack R M, Pírez G MC. [Cat-scratch disease with bone compromise: atypical manifestation].[Article in Spanish]. Rev Chilena Infectol. 2009 Aug;26(4):363-9. Epub 2009 Sep 23. PMID:19802407

Rolain JM, Boureau-Voultoury A, Raoult D. Serological evidence of Bartonella vinsonii lymphadenopathies in a child bitten by a dog. Clin Microbiol Infect. 2009 Dec;15 Suppl 2:122-3. Epub 2009 Apr 3. PMID:19374641

Rooks YL, Corwell B. Common urgent musculoskeletal injuries in primary care. Prim Care. 2006 Sep;33(3):751-77, viii. PMID:17088159

Rostoff P, Konduracka E, El Massri N, Gackowski A, Kruszec P, Zmudka K, Piwowarska W. [Lyme carditis presenting as acute coronary syndrome: a case report].[Article in Polish]. Kardiol Pol. 2008 Apr;66(4):420-5. PMID:18473271

Roubaud-Baudron C, Fortineau N, Goujard C, Le Bras P, Lambotte O. [Cat scratch disease with bone involvement: a case report and literature review].[Article in French]. Rev Med Interne. 2009 Jul;30(7):602-8. Epub 2009 Mar 19. PMID:19303175

Roux F, Boyer E, Jaulhac B, Dernis E, Closs-Prophette F, Puéchal X. Lyme meningoradiculitis: prospective evaluation of biological diagnosis methods. Eur J Clin Microbiol Infect Dis. 2007 Oct;26(10):685-93. PMID:17629757

Ruckenstein MJ, Prasthoffer A, Bigelow DC, Von Feldt JM, Kolasinski SL. Immunologic and serologic testing in patients with Ménière's disease. Otol Neurotol. 2002 Jul;23(4):517-20; discussion 520-1. PMID:12170155

Rudnik I, Konarzewska B, Zajkowska J, Juchnowicz D, Markowski T, Pancewicz SA. [The organic disorders in the course of Lyme disease]. [Article in Polish]. Pol Merkur Lekarski. 2004 Apr;16(94):328-31. PMID:15517926

Ruzić-Sabljić E, Maraspin V, Lotric-Furlan S, Jurca T, Logar M, Pikelj-Pecnik A, Strle F. Characterization of Borrelia burgdorferi sensu lato strains isolated from human material in Slovenia. Wien Klin Wochenschr. 2002 Jul 31;114(13-14):544-50. PMID:12422599

Saisongkorh W, Kowalczewska M, Azza S, Decloquement P, Rolain JM, Raoult D. Identification of candidate proteins for the diagnosis of Bartonella henselae infections using an immunoproteomic approach. FEMS Microbiol Lett. 2010 Sep 1;310(2):158-67. Epub 2010 Jul 9. PMID:20695898

Salehi N, Custodio H, Rathore MH. Renal microabscesses due to Bartonella infection. Pediatr Infect Dis J. 2010 May;29(5):472-3. PMID:20072078

Sanfeliu I, Antón E, Pineda V, Pons I, Perez J, Font B, Segura F. Description of Bartonella spp. infections in a general hospital of Catalonia, Spain. Clin Microbiol Infect. 2009 Dec;15 Suppl 2:130-1. Epub 2009 May 18. PMID:19456816

Sanguinetti-Morelli D, Angelakis E, Richet H, Davoust B, Rolain JM, Raoult D. Seasonality of cat-scratch disease, France, 1999-2009. Emerg Infect Dis. 2011 Apr;17(4):705-7. PMID:21470466

Sankatsing SU, Kolader ME, Bouma BJ, Bennink RJ, Verberne HJ, Ansink TM, Visser CE, van der Meer JT. 18F-fluoro-2-deoxyglucose positron emission tomography-negative endocarditis lenta caused by Bartonella henselae. J Heart Valve Dis. 2011 Jan;20(1):100-2. PMID:21404906

Sasseigne G, Herbert A, Larvol L, Damade R, Cartry O. [Fever and abdominal pain in a 56-year-old woman].[Article in French]. Rev Med Interne. 2009 Dec;30(12):1049-53. Epub 2009 Oct 7. PMID:19815317

Sauer A, Hansmann Y, Jaulhac B, Bourcier T, Speeg-Schatz C. [Ocular Lyme disease occurring during childhood: Five case reports.][Article in French]. J Fr Ophtalmol. 2011 Jun 20. [Epub ahead of print]. PMID:21696850

Scheidegger F, Quebatte M, Mistl C, Dehio C. The Bartonella henselae VirB/Bep system interferes with vascular endothelial growth factor (VEGF) signalling in human vascular endothelial cells. Cell Microbiol. 2011 Mar;13(3):419-31. Epub 2010 Dec 3. PMID:21044238

Schoen RT. A case revealing the natural history of untreated Lyme disease. Nat Rev Rheumatol. 2011 Mar;7(3):179-84. Epub 2010 Dec 21. PMID:21173795

Scott C, Azwa A, Cohen C, McIntyre M, Desmond N. Cat scratch disease: a diagnostic conundrum. Int J STD AIDS. 2009 Aug;20(8):585-6. PMID:19625597

Shah SS, Zaoutis TE, Turnquist J, Hodinka RL, Coffin SE. Early differentiation of Lyme from enteroviral meningitis. Pediatr Infect Dis J. 2005 Jun;24(6):542-5. PMID:15933566

Sherr VT. Panic attacks may reveal previously unsuspected chronic disseminated lyme disease. J Psychiatr Pract. 2000 Nov;6(6):352-6. PMID:15990495

Smajlovic F, Ibralic M. Color Doppler pseudolymphomatous manifestations of the cat scratch disease. Med Arh. 2009;63(5):297-9. PMID:20380135

Smismans A, Goossens VJ, Nulens E, Bruggeman CA. Comparison of five different immunoassays for the detection of Borrelia burgdorferi IgM and IgG antibodies. Clin Microbiol Infect. 2006 Jul;12(7):648-55. PMID:16774561

Steere AC, McHugh G, Damle N, Sikand VK. Prospective study of serologic tests for lyme disease. Clin Infect Dis. 2008 Jul 15;47(2):188-95. PMID:18532885

Stek CJ, van Eijk JJ, Jacobs BC, Enting RH, Sprenger HG, van Alfen N, van Assen S. Neuralgic amyotrophy associated with Bartonella henselae infection. J Neurol Neurosurg Psychiatry. 2011 Jun;82(6):707-8. Epub 2010 Aug 14. PMID:20710009

Stiles J. Bartonellosis in cats: a role in uveitis? Vet Ophthalmol. 2011 Sep;14 Suppl 1:9-14. PMID:21923819

Stone EG, Lacombe EH, Rand PW. Antibody testing and Lyme disease risk. Emerg Infect Dis. 2005 May;11(5):722-4. PMID:15890128

Stricker RB. Counterpoint: long-term antibiotic therapy improves persistent symptoms associated with lyme disease. Clin Infect Dis. 2007 Jul 15;45(2):149-57. Epub 2007 Jun 5. PMID:17578772

Stricker RB, Delong AK, Green CL, Savely VR, Chamallas SN, Johnson L. Benefit of intravenous antibiotic therapy in patients referred for treatment of neurologic Lyme disease. Int J Gen Med. 2011;4:639-46. Epub 2011 Sep 6. PMID:21941449

Stricker RB, Green CL, Savely VR, Chamallas SN, Johnson L. Safety of intravenous antibiotic therapy in patients referred for treatment of neurologic Lyme disease. Minerva Med. 2010 Feb;101(1):1-7. PMID:20228716

Stricker RB, Johnson L. Lyme wars: let's tackle the testing. BMJ. 2007 Nov 17;335(7628):1008. PMID:18006976

Stricker RB, Johnson L. Chronic Lyme disease and the 'Axis of Evil'. Future Microbiol. 2008 Dec;3(6):621-4. PMID:19072179

Stricker RB, Johnson L. Lyme disease: the next decade. Infect Drug Resist. 2011;4:1-9. Epub 2011 Jan 7. PMID:21694904

Strle F, Videcnik J, Zorman P, Cimperman J, Lotric-Furlan S, Maraspin V. Clinical and epidemiological findings for patients with erythema migrans. Comparison of cohorts from the years 1993 and 2000. Wien Klin Wochenschr. 2002 Jul 31;114(13-14):493-7. PMID:12422589

Stübs G, Fingerle V, Wilske B, Göbel UB, Zähringer U, Schumann RR, Schröder NW. Acylated cholesteryl galactosides are specific antigens of Borrelia causing lyme disease and frequently induce antibodies in late stages of disease. J Biol Chem. 2009 May 15;284(20):13326-34. Epub 2009 Mar 23. PMID:19307181

Sugiyama H, Sahara M, Imai Y, Ono M, Okamoto K, Kikuchi K, Nagai R. Infective endocarditis by Bartonella quintana masquerading as antineutrophil cytoplasmic antibody-associated small vessel vasculitis. Cardiology. 2009;114(3):208-11. Epub 2009 Jul 15. PMID:19602882

Suh B, Chun JK, Yong D, Lee YS, Jeong SH, Yang WI, Kim DS. A report of cat scratch disease in Korea confirmed by PCR amplification of the 16S-23S rRNA intergenic region of Bartonella henselae. Korean J Lab Med. 2010 Feb;30(1):34-7. PMID:20197720

Sun J, Fu G, Lin J, Song X, Lu L, Liu Q. Seroprevalence of Bartonella in Eastern China and analysis of risk factors. BMC Infect Dis. 2010 May 20;10:121. PMID:20482887

Sureda A, García D, Loma-Osorio P. [Embolic stroke as the first manifestation of Bartonella henselae endocarditis in an immunocompetent patient].[Article in Spanish]. Enferm Infecc Microbiol Clin. 2010 Jan;28(1):64-5. Epub 2009 May 1. PMID:19409676

Susta L, Uhl EW, Grosenbaugh DA, Krimer PM. Synovial Lesions in Experimental Canine Lyme Borreliosis. Vet Pathol. 2011 Nov 10. [Epub ahead of print]. PMID:22075774

Swanson SJ, Neitzel D, Reed KD, Belongia EA. Coinfections acquired from ixodes ticks. Clin Microbiol Rev. 2006 Oct;19(4):708-27. PMID:17041141

Sykes JE. Feline hemotropic mycoplasmas. J Vet Emerg Crit Care (San Antonio). 2010 Feb;20(1):62-9. PMID:20230435

Sykes JE, Lindsay LL, Maggi RG, Breitschwerdt EB. Human coinfection with Bartonella henselae and two hemotropic mycoplasma variants resembling Mycoplasma ovis. J Clin Microbiol. 2010 Oct;48(10):3782-5. Epub 2010 Aug 11. PMID:20702675

Sykes JE, Westropp JL, Kasten RW, Chomel BB. Association between Bartonella species infection and disease in pet cats as determined using serology and culture. J Feline Med Surg. 2010 Aug;12(8):631-6. Epub 2010 May 31. PMID:20570199

Szaleniec J, Oleś K, Składzień J, Strek P. [Cat scratch disease--an underestimated diagnosis].[Article in Polish]. Otolaryngol Pol. 2009 May-Jun;63(3):271-3. PMID:19886535

Talarek E, Duszczyk E, Zarnowska H. [Diagnostic difficulties in neuroborreliosis in children].[Article in Polish]/ Przegl Epidemiol. 2007;61(1):73-8. PMID:17702442

Tang YW. Duplex PCR assay simultaneously detecting and differentiating Bartonella quintana, B. henselae, and Coxiella burnetii in surgical heart valve specimens. J Clin Microbiol. 2009 Aug;47(8):2647-50. Epub 2009 Jun 24. PMID:19553582

Tarasów E, Ustymowicz A, Zajkowska J, Hermanowska-Szpakowicz T. [Neuroborreliosis: CT and MRI findings in 14 cases. Preliminary communication].[Article in Polish]. Neurol Neurochir Pol. 2001 Sep-Oct;35(5):803-13. PMID:11873593

Tasher D, Armarnik E, Mizrahi A, Liat BS, Constantini S, Grisaru-Soen G. Cat scratch disease with cervical vertebral osteomyelitis and spinal epidural abscess. Pediatr Infect Dis J. 2009 Sep;28(9):848-50. PMID:19654566

Tavora F, Burke A, Li L, Franks TJ, Virmani R. Postmortem confirmation of Lyme carditis with polymerase chain reaction. Cardiovasc Pathol. 2008 Mar-Apr;17(2):103-7. Epub 2007 May 11. PMID:18329555

Tay ST, Kamalanathan M, Rohani MY. Borrelia burgdorferi (strain B. afzelii) antibodies among Malaysian blood donors and patients. Southeast Asian J Trop Med Public Health. 2002 Dec;33(4):787-93. PMID:12757227

ten Hove CH, Gubler FM, Kiezebrink-Lindenhovius HH. Back pain in a child caused by cat scratch disease. Pediatr Infect Dis J. 2009 Mar;28(3):258. PMID:19209087

Teng JL, Yeung MY, Yue G, Au-Yeung RK, Yeung EY, Fung AM, Tse H, Yuen KY, Lau SK, Woo PC. In silico analysis of 16S rRNA gene sequencing based methods for identification of medically important aerobic Gram-negative bacteria. J Med Microbiol. 2011 Sep;60(Pt 9):1281-6. Epub 2011 Apr 15. PMID:21498652

Terekhova D, Sartakova ML, Wormser GP, Schwartz I, Cabello FC. Erythromycin resistance in Borrelia burgdorferi. Antimicrob Agents Chemother. 2002 Nov;46(11):3637-40. PMID:12384380

Terrada C, Bodaghi B, Conrath J, Raoult D, Drancourt M. Uveitis: an emerging clinical form of Bartonella infection. Clin Microbiol Infect. 2009 Dec;15 Suppl 2:132-3. Epub 2009 Jun 22. PMID:19548998

Thompson A, Mannix R, Bachur R. Acute pediatric monoarticular arthritis: distinguishing lyme arthritis from other etiologies. Pediatrics. 2009 Mar;123(3):959-65. PMID:19255026

Thompson GR 3rd, Lunetta JM, Johnson SM, Taylor S, Bays D, Cohen SH, Pappagianis D. Early treatment with fluconazole may abrogate the development of IgG antibodies in coccidioidomycosis. Clin Infect Dis. 2011 Sep;53(6):e20-4. PMID:21865185

Ticona E, Huaroto L, Garcia Y, Vargas L, Madariaga MG. The pathophysiology of the acute phase of human bartonellosis resembles AIDS. Med Hypotheses. 2010 Jan;74(1):45-9. Epub 2009 Aug 7. PMID:19665314

Tiemstra JD, Khatkhate N. Bell's palsy: diagnosis and management. Am Fam Physician. 2007 Oct 1;76(7):997-1002. PMID:17956069

Topolovec J, Puntarić D, Antolović-Pozgain A, Vuković D, Topolovec Z, Milas J, Drusko-Barisić V, Venus M. Serologically detected "new" tick-borne zoonoses in eastern Croatia. Croat Med J. 2003 Oct;44(5):626-9. PMID:14515426

Trafny DJ, Oyama MA, Wormser C, Reynolds CA, Singletary GE, Peddle GD. Cardiac troponin-I concentrations in dogs with bradyarrhythmias before and after artificial pacing. J Vet Cardiol. 2010 Dec;12(3):183-90. Epub 2010 Oct 28. PMID:21030328

Tsai YL, Chomel BB, Chang CC, Kass PH, Conrad PA, Chuang ST. Bartonella and Babesia infections in cattle and their ticks in Taiwan. Comp Immunol Microbiol Infect Dis. 2011 Mar;34(2):179-87. Epub 2010 Dec 30. PMID:21194750

Tsuneoka H, Yanagihara M, Otani S, Katayama Y, Fujinami H, Nagafuji H, Asari S, Nojima J, Ichihara K. A first Japanese case of Bartonella henselae-induced endocarditis diagnosed by prolonged culture of a specimen from the excised valve. Diagn Microbiol Infect Dis. 2010 Oct;68(2):174-6. PMID:20846591

Tuerlinckx D, Bodart E, Garrino MG, de Bilderling G. Clinical data and cerebrospinal fluid findings in Lyme meningitis versus aseptic meningitis. Eur J Pediatr. 2003 Mar;162(3):150-3. Epub 2003 Jan 21. PMID:12655417

Tuháčková J, Běláková J, Krupka M, Neperený J, Chumela J, Weigl E, Vrzal V. Testing of the Biocan B inj. ad us. vet. vaccine and development of the new recombinant vaccine against canine borreliosis. Biomed Pap Med Fac Univ Palacky Olomouc Czech Repub. 2005 Dec;149(2):297-302. PMID:16601776

Tylewska-Wierzbanowska S, Chmielewski T. Limitation of serological testing for Lyme borreliosis: evaluation of ELISA and western blot in comparison with PCR and culture methods. Wien Klin Wochenschr. 2002 Jul 31;114(13-14):601-5. PMID:12422608

Ullmann AJ, Gabitzsch ES, Schulze TL, Zeidner NS, Piesman J. Three multiplex assays for detection of Borrelia burgdorferi sensu lato and Borrelia miyamotoi sensu lato in field-collected Ixodes nymphs in North America. J Med Entomol. 2005 Nov;42(6):1057-62. PMID:16465748

Umekoji A, Fukai K, Yanagihara S, Ono E, Sowa J, Ishii M. Rapid detection of Bartonella henselae heat shock protein DNA by nested polymerase chain reaction from swollen lymph nodes of a patient with cat-scratch disease. J Dermatol. 2009 Oct;36(10):548-50. PMID:19785710

Valverde-Gubianas M, Ramos-López JF, López-Torres JA, Toribio-García M, Milla-Peñalver C, Gálvez Torres-Puchol J, Medialdea-Marcos S. [Neuroretinitis. Clinical cases].[Article in Spanish]. Arch Soc Esp Oftalmol. 2009 Aug;84(8):389-94. PMID:19728239

Varela AS, Luttrell MP, Howerth EW, Moore VA, Davidson WR, Stallknecht DE, Little SE. First culture isolation of Borrelia lonestari, putative agent of southern tick-associated rash illness. J Clin Microbiol. 2004 Mar;42(3):1163-9. PMID:15004069

Vayssier-Taussat M, Le Rhun D, Deng HK, Biville F, Cescau S, Danchin A, Marignac G, Lenaour E, Boulouis HJ, Mavris M, Arnaud L, Yang H, Wang J, Quebatte M, Engel P, Saenz H, Dehio C. The Trw type IV secretion system of Bartonella mediates host-specific adhesion to erythrocytes. PLoS Pathog. 2010 Jun 10;6(6):e1000946. PMID:20548954

Vázquez M, Sparrow SS, Shapiro ED. Long-term neuropsychologic and health outcomes of children with facial nerve palsy attributable to Lyme disease. Pediatrics. 2003 Aug;112(2):e93-7. PMID:12897313

Vermeulen MJ, Verbakel H, Notermans DW, Reimerink JH, Peeters MF. Evaluation of sensitivity, specificity and cross-reactivity in Bartonella henselae serology. J Med Microbiol. 2010 Jun;59(Pt 6):743-5. Epub 2010 Mar 11. PMID:20223899

Vianello M, Marchiori G, Giometto B. Multiple cranial nerve involvement in Bannwarth's syndrome. Neurol Sci. 2008 Apr;29(2):109-12. Epub 2008 May 16. PMID:18483708

Vitale G, Incandela S, Incandela C, Micalizzi A, Mansueto P. Isolation and characterization of Bartonella quintana from the parotid gland of an immunocompetent man. J Clin Microbiol. 2009 Mar;47(3):862-4. Epub 2009 Jan 7. PMID:19129406

Vorstman JA, Kuiper H. [Peripheral facial palsy in children: test for lyme borreliosis only in the presence of other clinical signs].[Article in Dutch]. Ned Tijdschr Geneeskd. 2004 Apr 3;148(14):655-8. PMID:15106315

Vostal K, Zakovska A. Two-year study of examination of blood from wild rodents for the presence of antiborrelian antibodies. Ann Agric Environ Med. 2003;10(2):203-6. PMID:14677912

Wagner B, Freer H, Rollins A, Erb HN. A fluorescent bead-based multiplex assay for the simultaneous detection of antibodies to B. burgdorferi outer surface proteins in canine serum. Vet Immunol Immunopathol. 2011 Apr 15;140(3-4):190-8. Epub 2010 Dec 10. PMID:21208663

Wagner B, Freer H, Rollins A, Erb HN, Lu Z, Gröhn Y. Development of a multiplex assay for the detection of antibodies to Borrelia burgdorferi in horses and its validation using Bayesian and conventional statistical methods. Vet Immunol Immunopathol. 2011 Dec 15;144(3-4):374-81. Epub 2011 Aug 17. PMID:21890217

Wang CW, Chang WC, Chao TK, Liu CC, Huang GS. Computed tomography and magnetic resonance imaging of cat-scratch disease: a report of two cases. Clin Imaging. 2009 Jul-Aug;33(4):318-21. PMID:19559357

Webster JD, Miller MA, DuSold D, Ramos-Vara J. Effects of prolonged formalin fixation on the immunohistochemical detection of infectious agents in formalin-fixed, paraffin-embedded tissues. Vet Pathol. 2010 May;47(3):529-35. Epub 2010 Mar 23. PMID:20332424

Weinspach S, Tenenbaum T, Schönberger S, Schaper J, Engers R, Rueggeberg J, Mackenzie CR, Wolf A, Mayatepek E, Schroten H. Cat scratch disease--heterogeneous in clinical presentation: five unusual cases of an infection caused by Bartonella henselae. Klin Padiatr. 2010 Mar;222(2):73-8. Epub 2009 Sep 29. PMID:19790029

Weinstein A. Editorial commentary: laboratory testing for Lyme disease: time for a change? Clin Infect Dis. 2008 Jul 15;47(2):196-7. PMID:18532894

Welc-Faleciak R. [Current state of the knowledge of Bartonella infections].[Article in Polish]. Przegl Epidemiol. 2009;63(1):11-7. PMID:19522219

Welc-Faleciak R, Rodo A, Siński E, Bajer A. Babesia canis and other tick-borne infections in dogs in Central Poland. Vet Parasitol. 2009 Dec 23;166(3-4):191-8. Epub 2009 Sep 26. PMID:19837515

Wendling D, Sevrin P, Bouchaud-Chabot A, Chabroux A, Toussirot E, Bardin T, Michel F. Parsonage-Turner syndrome revealing Lyme borreliosis. Joint Bone Spine. 2009 Mar;76(2):202-4. Epub 2009 Jan 14. PMID:19147387

Woodcock S. Lyme disease testing. Lancet Infect Dis. 2006 Mar;6(3):122. PMID:16500588

Wormser GP, Liveris D, Hanincová K, Brisson D, Ludin S, Stracuzzi VJ, Embers ME, Philipp MT, Levin A, Aguero-Rosenfeld M, Schwartz I. Effect of Borrelia burgdorferi genotype on the sensitivity of C6 and 2-tier testing in North American patients with culture-confirmed Lyme disease. Clin Infect Dis. 2008 Oct 1;47(7):910-4. PMID:18724824

Wormser GP, Nowakowski J, Nadelman RB, Visintainer P, Levin A, Aguero-Rosenfeld E. Impact of clinical variables on Borrelia burgdorferi-specific antibody seropositivity in acute-phase sera from patients in North America with culture-confirmed early Lyme disease. Clin Vaccine Immunol. 2008 Oct;15(10):1519-22. Epub 2008 Aug 20. PMID:18716009

Wormser GP, Ramanathan R, Nowakowski J, McKenna D, Holmgren D, Visintainer P, Dornbush R, Singh B, Nadelman RB. Duration of antibiotic therapy for early Lyme disease. A randomized, double-blind, placebo-controlled trial. Ann Intern Med. 2003 May 6;138(9):697-704. PMID:12729423

Wright SA, Tucker JR, Donohue AM, Castro MB, Kelley KL, Novak MG, Macedo PA. Avian hosts of Ixodes pacificus (Acari: Ixodidae) and the detection of Borrelia burgdorferi in larvae feeding on the Oregon junco. J Med Entomol. 2011 Jul;48(4):852-9. PMID:21845945

Yamada Y, Ohkusu K, Yanagihara M, Tsuneoka H, Ezaki T, Tsuboi J, Okabayashi H, Suwabe A. Prosthetic valve endocarditis caused by Bartonella quintana in a patient during immunosuppressive therapies for collagen vascular diseases. Diagn Microbiol Infect Dis. 2011 Jul;70(3):395-8. Epub 2011 May 10. PMID:21558050

Yilmaz C, Ergin C, Kaleli I. [Investigation of Bartonella henselae seroprevalence and related risk factors in blood donors admitted to Pamukkale University Blood Center].[Article in Turkish]. Mikrobiyol Bul. 2009 Jul;43(3):391-401. PMID:19795614

Yoon HJ, Lee WC, Choi YS, Cho S, Song YG, Choi JY, Kim CO, Kim EJ, Kim JM. Cervical lymphadenitis in a patient coinfected with Toxoplasma gondii and Bartonella henselae. Vector Borne Zoonotic Dis. 2010 May;10(4):415-9. PMID:19874186

Youssef D, Shams WE, El Abbassi A, Moorman JP, Al-Abbadi MA. Combining cytomorphology and serology for the diagnosis of cat scratch disease. Diagn Cytopathol. 2011 Mar;39(3):210-3. PMID:21319324

Zajkowska JM, Hermanowska-Szpakowicz T, Wysocka J, Pancewicz S, Lipska A, Kasprzycka E. [Estimation of platelet counts and their morphological parameters in patients infected by borrelia burgdorferi].[Article in Polish]. Wiad Lek. 2001;54(11-12):668-73. PMID:11928555

Zapater Latorre E, Castillo Ruiz A, Alba García JR, Armengot Carceller M, Sancho Rieger J, Basterra Alegría J. [Bilateral peripheral facial paralysis secondary to Lyme disease].[Article in Spanish]. An Otorrinolaringol Ibero Am. 2004;31(5):447-58. PMID:15566265

Zarraga M, Rosen L, Herschthal D. Bacillary angiomatosis in an immunocompetent child: a case report and review of the literature. Am J Dermatopathol. 2011 Jul;33(5):513-5. PMID:21285862

Zarzycka B, Pieczara A, Skowron-Kobos J, Krzemiński Z. [Prevalence IgG antibodies against Bartonella henselae in children with lymphadenopathy].[Article in Polish]. Przegl Epidemiol. 2008;62(4):759-65. PMID:19209738

Zeidner NS, Schneider BS, Dolan MC, Piesman J. An analysis of spirochete load, strain, and pathology in a model of tick-transmitted Lyme borreliosis. Vector Borne Zoonotic Dis. 2001 Spring;1(1):35-44. PMID:12653134

Zenone T. Systemic Bartonella henselae Infection in Immunocompetent Adult Presenting as Fever of Unknown Origin. Case Report Med. 2011;2011:183937. Epub 2011 May 5. PMID:21629850

Zekraoui Y, Megzari A, El Alloussi T, Berraho A. [Unilateral neuroretinitis revealing cat-scratch disease].[Article in French]. Rev Med Interne. 2011 Apr;32(4):e46-8. Epub 2010 Jun 19. PMID:20646795

Zhang L, Cui F, Wang L, Zhang L, Zhang J, Wang S, Yang S. Investigation of anaplasmosis in Yiyuan County, Shandong Province, China. Asian Pac J Trop Med. 2011 Jul;4(7):568-72. PMID:21803311

Zhong J, Skouloubris S, Dai Q, Myllykallio H, Barbour AG. Function and evolution of plasmid-borne genes for pyrimidine biosynthesis in Borrelia spp. J Bacteriol. 2006 Feb;188(3):909-18. PMID:16428394

Zobba R, Chessa G, Mastrandrea S, Pinna Parpaglia ML, Patta C, Masala G. Serological and molecular detection of Bartonella spp. in humans, cats and dogs from northern Sardinia, Italy. Clin Microbiol Infect. 2009 Dec;15 Suppl 2:134-5. Epub 2009 May 18. PMID:19456814

The Babesia Checklist

Improving Detection of A Common, Emerging Stealth Infection

James L. Schaller, M.D., M.A.R.

Introduction

Below are examples of signs, symptoms and indirect ways to help increase the diagnosis of Babesia. An examination of public genetic databases shows that well over thirty-five species exist, many of which have variants.

Please note that an unknown percentage of people infected with this single celled parasite have no symptoms, at least for many years.

This checklist is not meant to be used as a definitive tool to diagnose Babesia.   It is my expert opinion that no definitive 100% or even 98% accurate tool exists.

My goal is merely to decrease illness in those people who are positive but do not show up as positive on a basic direct test (false negative).

Indeed, it is not uncommon for a patient with Babesia to present with a negative test result over ten times, regardless of the laboratory, and then to show up with a positive on DNA testing when exposed to two or three treatments against protozoa for three days, or to have new conversion from negative to positive antibody testing six weeks after a similar provocation trial.

I do not oppose or endorse such approaches, but feel it necessary to mention that the same outcome has occurred with "Malaria- prevention" treatment. Additionally, there have been instances in which the use of herbs, such as artesunate, for cancer prevention, has resulted in an unintended outcome: the conversion of a Babesia antibody titer from negative to positive.

Having authored four books on the topic of Babesia, I have created this scale based on years of full-time reading and a passion to advance detection.   This checklist is meant to prevent false negatives: some patients who appear to be negative may not actually be negative. I have done this because my years of full-time reading and research have shown me that missing this parasite for 5, 10, 30 or 50 years is far more dangerous than careful treatment. Treatment side effects are low if the treatment is started at **20% of the suggested dose.**

I would appeal to you that one cannot be considered an expert in treating this potentially fatal infection by merely reading a few articles or guidelines. Nor is expertise acquired by diagnosing and treating the highly obvious, immensely ill, sickest 1% of patients as the "norm" in Babesia diagnosis. Expertise should require *at least* a review of 1500 articles over five years. The fact that parasite textbooks usually offer merely 1-2 pages about this infection shows that it is not mastered or understood even by those interested in parasites.

The cure of Babesia does not fit a set formula, but no one should be hopeless about reaching a full recovery. I have currently started a new, research-based, creative thinking textbook on **optimal Babesia treatments** for publication in 2012. It will discuss familiar treatments and offer ideas to maximize these options, but I will also add discussions on newer options for patients and clinicians who are not satisfied with the current options.

In summary, how can any certain medical or scientific Babesia position exist, when new species, sub-species or variants that infect humans are routinely emerging, and for which there is not even a direct test— regardless of sensitivity?

THE BABESIA CHECKLIST

James Schaller, M.D., M.A.R.

(Please Check Any Symptoms That Apply)

PSYCHIATRIC AND NEUROLOGICAL

☐ Family, friends or others report you look tired or foggy

☐ Slowed thinking

☐ Psychiatric label(s) given to a child or relative for all their troubles when clear medical problems exist as shown by abnormal laboratory results (I am not talking about basic organ failure labs, but the use of *wide testing which includes inflammation and anti-inflammation chemicals, hormones, nutrient levels, and other immune system chemicals*)

☐ Enlarged lymph nodes (but also in Lyme, Bartonella, other infections, high inflammation, tumors and other diseases)

☐ Brain troubles such as trouble keeping up with past routine life demands, lateness due to trouble with motivation and organization, and trouble with concentration [Any of these would be a positive]

☐ Memory troubles [this is not specific to one infection or one disease process.   For example, exposure to indoor mold's biological chemicals can decrease memory within an hour depending on the species mix.]

☐ Profound psychiatric illnesses [this is not limited to a single infection.]

HEART & CIRCULATORY SYSTEM

☐ A sudden loss of blood pressure

☐ Transfusions using blood that is not your own

☐ Anemia even if a non-infectious cause has been proposed

☐ Anemia without a clear explanation

☐ Severe chest wall pains

☐ A "heart attack" before the age of 55 (when you have three risk factors)

☐ A "heart attack" or infarct of the heart before the age of 60 years old, with only one risk factor.   [Being male is **considered** a risk factor for many.   Men **experience** heart damage sooner than women.   Other risk factors include tobacco use or exposure, such as second hand smoke at home, diabetes, high blood pressure, high level of sticky cholesterol such as Lipoprotein (a) or high triglyceride levels, family history of heart attacks, limited physical activity, Obesity (might be defined as wearing pants over 39 inches if you are a man and over 34 inches if you a woman or a body fat or body mass index of 30 or higher), excess anger or routine poor handling of stress, and abuse of stimulant drugs such as cocaine or amphetamines. I would add a homocysteine laboratory level over 10, major depression, no vitamin K2 supplementation, a free dihydrotestosterone in the 10th percentile or lower, fragmented or poor sleep [which increases inflammation], a high C4a RIA, a MMPI in excess of 300 and a low VIP blood level.

MAJOR ORGANS

☐ A yellow hue on eyes, hands and skin (jaundice) with no other clear cause

☐ An enlarged liver (which sits under your right rib cage)

☐ An enlarged spleen (under your left rib cage).   **This is falsely believed to be a common human sign; actually it is very rare.**

☐ A ruptured spleen [rare but it gets fast medical attention and therefore is over-represented in medical articles]

☐ Dark urine [this is rarer than some articles intimate]

☐ An inability to urinate

☐ Shortness of breath [no clear asthma, pneumonia, COPD or other common cause]

☐ Pulmonary edema which is a high amount of fluid in the air sacs of the lungs, which leads to shortness of breath

☐ A stroke of any size or in any organ (the word stroke means tissue is unable to get oxygen). The stroke or infarct can be in the brain, retina, kidney, heart and many other tissues.

☐ An MRI, CT or other imaging study that shows dead tissue in any organ with no known cause

GENERAL MEDICAL

☐ Headaches with no clear cause

☐ Headaches which are hard to control and/or severe

☐ Headaches lasting over three years and which increase in pain despite treatments

☐ Weight gain in clear excess of diet and exercise

☐ Weight loss with reasonable eating and average exercise

☐ Excess fat in lower belly area that is in excess of lifestyle and activity

☐ Anorexia or a decrease in appetite

☐ Any decrease in appetite

☐ A poor appetite

☐ Fatigue in excess of that experienced by most people in the same age range

☐ Fatigue that produces need for sleep in excess of 8 ½ hours daily

☐ Fatigue with ongoing insomnia [consider the possibility of both Bartonella and Babesia in this case]

☐ Daytime sleep urgency despite nighttime sleep

☐ Night sweats

☐ Excessive perspiration during normal daily activity

☐ Hot flashes in a normal temperature room

☐ Intermittent fever

☐ Chills

☐ Any fever in excess of three days

☐ Spike of a fever over 100.5 after a possible tick bite

☐ Listlessness

☐ Swelling in limbs and other parts of body

☐ Waves of generalized itching [this sign of infection and inflammation is not limited just to Babesia.]

☐ Lumps or other types of tissue collection with no clear cause [Other tick and flea-borne infections can also cause these growths.]

☐ Wasting muscles

☐ The general wasting away of body tissue that is visible

☐ Profound bone loss in marked excess of that **expected at given age**

☐ Excess breast tissue in a man or boy

☐ Random stabbing pains

☐ Nausea or vomiting

☐ Any enhanced sense: sensitivity to light, touch, smells, taste or sound

☐ A sense of imbalance

☐ One or more medical problems with unclear cause(s), with changing or contradictory diagnoses, or which are eventually called "idiopathic"

☐ Two tick or flea infections with two positive tick or flea-borne viruses, bacteria or protozoa.   The presence of other infections such as tick-borne viruses or bacteria raises suspicion of a Babesia infection.

☐ The presence of one or more mystery illnesses after an evaluation by three quality physicians

LAB RESULTS

☐ Eosinophil Cationic Protein (ECP) level is in top 15% of normal. This is altered in perhaps 15-20% of Babesia patients.

☐ The ECP level is above normal.   (Other things can increase this lab, but it is an error that a Babesia infection is not on these lists).

☐ The ECP level increases 30% or more in response to a protozoa killing medication in serial testing.   (This test is about 40-60% sensitive and many patients have no change in this lab even with effective treatment).

☐ The ECP level is below detectable levels.

☐ Absolute Eosinophils in the low or high range [this is not definitive in any manner, but is a useful tool.]

☐ A percentage of Eosinophils in low range or high normal range

☐ Very high Eosinophils [rare with Babesia, but other findings suggest other possible causes]

☐   A normal or low VEGF lab result in the presence of Bartonella

☐   A TNF-alpha in excess of 1.0 in the presence of Bartonella

☐   A CD57 or CD57/8 level that drops right after the start of a Babesia treatment, or which falls steadily with ongoing Babesia treatment

☐   Hemolytic anemia with lab test showing positive blood products in your urine [this is not a routine finding.]

☐   Your clinician understands the use of indirect testing and feels your lab pattern is suggestive of the presence of Babesia.   This involves more than an ECP spike.

☐   Since direct testing for Babesia by any lab misses many human species and is of variable reliability, and the common presence of Bartonella suppresses some antibody tests, a positive or "indeterminate" is likely a positive.   Have you had an "indeterminate" or "borderline" Babesia result?

☐   Bilirubin abnormality [elevated in perhaps 5 % of patients]

☐   Iron abnormalities in excess of normal [high or low levels. The finding of genetic disease that increases iron pathology does not necessarily rule out this finding.   The iron pathology can be genetic or acquired illness plus Babesia [See my HES cancer cure paper in Medscape in which the cancer-like eosinophils were primed by Babesia].

☐   After Babesia treatment with clear protozoa killing agents used also to kill malaria, IL-6 moves from very low to an increased level.

☐   After Babesia treatment with clear protozoa killing agents used also to kill malaria, IL-1B moves from very low to an increased level.

☐ Babesia creates and provokes changes in the human body chemistry. Tests are being designed to identify chemicals only made by Babesia. A sample is Babesia microti secreted antigen 1 (BmSA1).

☐ Any positive Epstein-Barr virus over the normal low level. You may have an infection, infections, or inflammation. It is not merely found in Babesia. [This is not a routine cause of fatigue].

☐ Autoimmunity testing is positive. This is a stronger positive if there are two autoimmune results. For example, a patient has a positive ANA and has antibodies against their thyroid system.

☐ Positive lab or skin testing placing patient's food sensitivity in top 5% of population

☐ Elevated monocytes

☐ Elevated neutrophils with no clear infection source

☐ Elevated C-reactive protein

☐ Elevated D-dimer

☐ An abnormally high ALT which is a liver enzyme increased by liver trauma, toxins or infections such as Babesia [a rare finding].

☐ Lymphocytopenia—low lymphocytes which are a type of infection-fighting white blood cell

☐ Thrombocytopenia—platelet number under 50,000

☐ A high lactate dehydrogenase or LDH. This enzyme measures tissue damage particularly found in the heart, liver, kidney, skeletal muscle, brain, blood cells and lungs.

REACTION OR CHANGES IN BODY

☐ React to any derivative of Artemisia (Sweet Wormwood). *Note: the reaction does not need to last more than a day and any immediate stomachaches or loose stools do not apply.

☐ React to a malaria drug.   For example, ativoquone (Mepron), proguanil alone or with ativoquone (Malarone), artesunate, day 1-3 of artemesinin, a new high dose of artemesinin Day 1-2, artemeter, Alinia, clindamycin, quinine or azithromycin at 2,000 mg/day orally or at any dose IV for five straight days.   (It requires profound wisdom for a clinician to distinguish between a side effect and a reaction caused by an effective Babesia treatment.   For example, insomnia caused by the synthetic drug Larium is meaningless, since Larium has this as a side effect in uninfected patients.   But fatigue, insomnia or severe headache resulting from a teaspoon of ativoquone (Mepron) on day one are very suspicious symptoms for a known protozoan like Babesia or Malaria or other similar infections that are newly identified genetically).

☐ Mood changes with any herb or drug that kills protozoa like Babesia, with the exception of Larium

☐ Muscle aches or joint aches/pain, especially worse after use of a protozoa killing medicine such as proquanil, Alinia, ativoquone, clindamycin, or one of many new emerging progressive natural medicine or synthetic malaria drug treatments

☐ Insomnia after taking a malaria killing herb or drug

☐ Anxiety and/or depression after taking a malaria killing herb or drug

☐ Rage or temporary personality regression right after use of a malaria killing herb or medication, e.g., ativoquone, Malarone, proguanil, artesunate, day 1-3 of artemesinin, artemeter, Alinia, clindamycin or azithromycin at 2,000 mg/day orally or at any dose IV for five straight days.

ENVIRONMENT

☐ Pets, farm animals or local relatives with ANY **clinical symptoms** of a tick-borne virus, bacteria or protozoa infection without a clear diagnosis

☐ The patient's **mother** is suspected of having or has been diagnosed with Babesia, STARI (Masterson's Disease), Neoehrlichia, Anaplasma, Lyme disease, Mycoplasmas, Q Fever, Rocky Mountain spotted fever (Rickettsia), tick-borne relapsing fever, Tularemia (bacteria), Ehrlichia, Protozoa FL1953, or viruses such as CMV, HHV-6, Coxsackie B Types 1, 2, 3, 4, 5, 6, Parvo B-19 or Powassan.

☐ **A sibling, father, spouse or child** with any tick borne infection who shared a residence or vacation with proximity to brush (wooded area)

☐ Exposure to outdoor environments with brush, wild grasses, wild streams, golf courses or woods *in excess of ten minutes in any location lived in or visited*

☐ **Pet(s) or family animals** of any type, e.g., horses, have had outdoor exposures to areas with brush, wild grasses, wild streams or woods.   If the pets were animals such as dogs, which can be given anti-tick and flea treatments, were these animals always *on schedule* with these treatments?

☐ Clear exposure to ticks in your current or past homes

☐ Clear exposure to ticks during vacations or other travels

☐ Have you ever had any type of tick bite?

☐ Have you ever found a tick on your clothing?

☐ Have you ever found a tick on your body?

☐ Have you been with others at a location in which they had ticks on their clothing or skin?

☐ Sexual contact is a debated form of communication of some tick and flea borne infections.   I have no position.   Isolation in a body fluid does not mean that is a route to spread the infection. If you and your healer feel this is a possible route of infection, has the patient had intimate contact with the sharing of body fluids with an infected person?

☐ You live in a state that has reports of any tick-borne infection in over 40 people.   [Currently, this would usually be Lyme disease only].

☐ You live next to a state that has reports of any tick-borne infection in over 60 people.   [Currently, this would usually be Lyme disease only].

☐ Many small mammals live near your home, exercise location, vacation locations or work.

A WORD ON MANUAL BLOOD EXAMINATIONS

No blood smear will be positive for Babesia unless you have a profound number of infected red blood cells.   This is very rare.   Therefore, **no blood smear should be considered negative unless it has been examined for at least thirty minutes.**   While a 2-3 minute exam of large white blood cells may be fully sufficient to identify cancers and other diseases, a search for over eighty Babesia red blood cell presentations under 1000x, as found in my book, *Hematology Forms of Babesia,* requires at least thirty minutes.   Unfortunately, in patients positive for Babesia, routine manual red blood smear exams with a clear request to look for Babesia under a microscope at 1,000x magnification have missed the Babesia at least 98% of the time.   In papers reporting clearly visualized Babesia in blood smears the patients tend to have immense infection, i.e., over 3% of red blood cells are infected.

However, if one privately contracts with a microbiologist, pathologist or can get a lab director to allow their staff to spend the extra time, the positive results on the blood smear increase with clearly positively infected patients.   I know most laboratories are very overworked, but the notion that a blood slide is going to show an obvious tetrad or a classic X pattern is an error.   Using slides from respected national or state sources, I found only by very careful exam, over fifty presentations of Babesia that are usually missed.   Indeed, in my textbook on Babesia images most of the shapes had never been published.   No one in history had ever taken the time to look carefully at 200 slides and record each unique shape.   It is fairly stunning to write this and confirms that many tick and flea infections are clearly emerging and not yet mastered.

Please appreciate that stains help define whether a substance is what it appears to be.   For example, some in the alternative medicine school feel that Candida is a bad presence in the intestines and feel it often gets into the blood through defects in the intestinal wall.   While Candida is not a good presence for the intestine, I have found that some blood samples with items that look significantly like parts of Candida do not stain for cellulose and other components of yeasts.   My point is that in the last ten years, in discussions or study, excellent pathologists and microbiologists have shown me the clear reason humanity has developed highly sophisticated staining techniques--they can be diagnostic and very cost effective.   And some medical scientists are adding new technology to Babesia identification (discussed in my *Babesia 2009 Update* and my *Hematology of Babesia* text).

Babesia is an emerging infection.   Any certainty claims or criticism about Babesia positions without extensive research and over 200 hours of reading is premature.   Again, new Babesia species are emerging every one to four months.   Indeed, even a new protozoan has been found that looks like Babesia under a high powered microscope, but when it is genetically sequenced it is not Babesia or immature malaria, which can look similar.   It is a new infection and is presently called FL1953 and was genetically sequenced by Dr. Ellis and Dr. Fry. It looks like Babesia, but is not Babesia genetically.

Therefore, since human Babesia is a new emerging illness, this scale is meant merely to increase awareness of Babesia, an infection that can kill patients of any age.   Writings in the past fifteen years have either seen Babesia as a mere "co-infection" or a footnote of a spirochete infection [i.e., Lyme].   Anything that can hide for a couple of decades, and then possibly kill you with a clot in your heart, brain or lungs or by other means, is not a casual infection.

Babesia cure claims should be made with the use of indirect testing birthed from extracts of superior journals read a minimum of five years. Currently, these many well-established indirect lab test patterns are not used or understood by immensely busy and smart clinicians working full-time. While this is fully understandable, I hope it may change in the coming decade.

Dr. Schaller is the author of 30 books and 27 top journal articles. His publications address issues in at least twelve fields of medicine.

He has published the most recent four textbooks on Babesia.

He has published on Babesia as a cancer primer under the supervision of the former editor of the *Journal of the American Medical Association (JAMA)*, and his entries on multiple tick and flea-borne infections, including Babesia [along with Bartonella and Lyme disease], were published in a respected infection textbook endorsed by the NIH Director of Infectious Disease.

Dr. Schaller has produced seven texts on tick and flea-borne infections based on his markedly unique full-time reading and study practice, which is not limited to either finite traditional or integrative progressive medicine. With a physician's medical license, he has been able to sort through many truth claims by ordering lab testing. He does not casually follow the dozens of yearly truth claims, without indirect testing laboratory proof. He has read full-time on these emerging problems for many years. He is rated a TOP and BEST physician (in the top 5 percent of doctors) by both physician peers and patients.

Bibliography (Babesia)

Abbas HM, Brenes RA, Ajemian MS, Scholand SJ. Successful conservative treatment of spontaneous splenic rupture secondary to Babesiosis: a case report and literature review. Conn Med. 2011 Mar;75(3):143-6. PMID:21500704

AbouLaila M, Sivakumar T, Yokoyama N, Igarashi I. Inhibitory effect of terpene nerolidol on the growth of Babesia parasites. Parasitol Int. 2010 Jun;59(2):278-82. Epub 2010 Feb 21. PMID:20178862

Aderinboye O, Syed SS. Congenital babesiosis in a four-week-old female infant. Pediatr Infect Dis J. 2010 Feb;29(2):188. PMID:20118748

Alekseev AN. [The possibility of the detection of one more tick-borne infection--babesiosis--on the territory of Russia].[Article in Russian]. Zh Mikrobiol Epidemiol Immunobiol. 2003 May-Jun;(3):39-43. PMID:12886630

Alekseev AN, Rudakov NV, Dubinina EV. [Possible types of tick-borne diseases and the predictive role of history data in their diagnosis (parasitological aspects of the problem)].[Article in Russian]. Med Parazitol (Mosk). 2004 Oct-Dec;(4):31-6. PMID:15689134

Alkhalil A, Hill DA, Desai SA. Babesia and plasmodia increase host erythrocyte permeability through distinct mechanisms. Cell Microbiol. 2007 Apr;9(4):851-60. Epub 2006 Nov 3. PMID:17087736

Arai S, Tsuji M, Kaiho I, Murayama H, Zamoto A, Wei Q, Okabe N, Kamiyama T, Ishihara C. Retrospective seroepidemiological survey for human babesiosis in an area in Japan where a tick-borne disease is endemic. J Vet Med Sci. 2003 Mar;65(3):335-40. PMID:12679563

Armstrong PM, Brunet LR, Spielman A, Telford SR 3rd. Risk of Lyme disease: perceptions of residents of a Lone Star tick-infested community. Bull World Health Organ. 2001;79(10):916-25. PMID:11693973

Arnez M, Luznik-Bufon T, Avsic-Zupanc T, Ruzic-Sabljic E, Petrovec M, Lotric-Furlan S, Strle F. Causes of febrile illnesses after a tick bite in Slovenian children. Pediatr Infect Dis J. 2003 Dec;22(12):1078-83. PMID:14688569

Asad S, Sweeney J, Mermel LA. Transfusion-transmitted babesiosis in Rhode Island. Transfusion. 2009 Dec;49(12):2564-73. Epub 2009 Sep 16. PMID:19761547

Babu RV, Sharma G. A 57-year-old man with abdominal pain, jaundice, and a history of blood transfusion. Chest. 2007 Jul;132(1):347-50. PMID:17625097

Barratt JL, Harkness J, Marriott D, Ellis JT, Stark D. Importance of nonenteric protozoan infections in immunocompromised people. Clin Microbiol Rev. 2010 Oct;23(4):795-836. PMID:20930074

Baumann D, Pusterla N, Péter O, Grimm F, Fournier PE, Schär G, Bossart W, Lutz H, Weber R. [Fever after a tick bite: clinical manifestations and diagnosis of acute tick bite-associated infections in northeastern Switzerland]. [Article in German] Dtsch Med Wochenschr. 2003 May 9;128(19):1042-7. PMID:12736854

Baumeister S, Wiesner J, Reichenberg A, Hintz M, Bietz S, Harb OS, Roos DS, Kordes M, Friesen J, Matuschewski K, Lingelbach K, Jomaa H, Seeber F. Fosmidomycin uptake into Plasmodium and Babesia-infected erythrocytes is facilitated by parasite-induced new permeability pathways. PLoS One. 2011 May 4;6(5):e19334. PMID:21573242

Belongia EA, Reed KD, Mitchell PD, Mueller-Rizner N, Vandermause M, Finkel MF, Kazmierczak JJ. Tickborne infections as a cause of nonspecific febrile illness in Wisconsin. Clin Infect Dis. 2001 May 15;32(10):1434-9. Epub 2001 Apr 17. PMID:11317244

Birkenheuer AJ, Whittington J, Neel J, Large E, Barger A, Levy MG, Breitschwerdt

EB. Molecular characterization of a Babesia species identified in a North American raccoon. J Wildl Dis. 2006 Apr;42(2):375-80. PMID:16870860

Blue D, Graves V, McCarthy L, Cruz J, Gregurek S, Smith D. Fatal transfusion-transmitted Babesia microti in the Midwest. Transfusion. 2009 Jan;49(1):8. Epub 2008 Aug 6. PMID:18694463

Braga W, Venasco J, Willard L, Moro MH. Ultrastructure of Babesia WA1 (Apicomplexa: Piroplasma) during infection of erythrocytes in a hamster model. J Parasitol. 2006 Oct;92(5):1104-7. PMID:17152960

Breitschwerdt EB, Maggi RG. A confusing case of canine vector-borne disease: clinical signs and progression in a dog co-infected with Ehrlichia canis and Bartonella vinsonii ssp. berkhoffii. Parasit Vectors. 2009 Mar 26;2 Suppl 1:S3. PMID:19426442

Brigden ML. Detection, education and management of the asplenic or hyposplenic patient. Am Fam Physician. 2001 Feb 1;63(3):499-506, 508. PMID:11272299

Buelvas F, Alvis N, Buelvas I, Miranda J, Mattar S. [A high prevalence of antibodies against Bartonella and Babesia microti has been found in villages and urban populations in Cordoba, Colombia].[Article in Spanish]. Rev Salud Publica (Bogota). 2008 Jan-Feb;10(1):168-77. PMID:18368229

Cacciò S, Cammà C, Onuma M, Severini C. The beta-tubulin gene of Babesia and Theileria parasites is an informative marker for species discrimination. Int J Parasitol. 2000 Oct;30(11):1181-5. PMID:11027785

Cangelosi JJ, Sarvat B, Sarria JC, Herwaldt BL, Indrikovs AJ. Transmission of Babesia microti by blood transfusion in Texas. Vox Sang. 2008 Nov;95(4):331-4. PMID:19138264

Cardoso L, Tuna J, Vieira L, Yisaschar-Mekuzas Y, Baneth G. Molecular detection of Anaplasma platys and Ehrlichia canis in dogs from the North of Portugal. Vet J. 2010 Feb;183(2):232-3. Epub 2008 Dec 3. PMID:19056304

Carter WJ, Yan Z, Cassai ND, Sidhu GS. Detection of extracellular forms of babesia in the blood by electron microscopy: a diagnostic method for differentiation from Plasmodium falciparum. Ultrastruct Pathol. 2003 Jul-Aug;27(4):211-6. PMID:12907365

Centeno-Lima S, do Rosário V, Parreira R, Maia AJ, Freudenthal AM, Nijhof AM, Jongejan F. A fatal case of human babesiosis in Portugal: molecular and phylogenetic analysis. Trop Med Int Health. 2003 Aug;8(8):760-4. PMID:12869099

Chatel G, Gulletta M, Matteelli A, Marangoni A, Signorini L, Oladeji O, Caligaris S. Short report: Diagnosis of tick-borne relapsing fever by the quantitative buffy coat fluorescence method. Am J Trop Med Hyg. 1999 May;60(5):738-9. PMID:10344644

Cichocka A, Skotarczak B. [Babesosis--difficulty of diagnosis].[Article in Polish]. Wiad Parazytol. 2001;47(3):527-33. PMID:16894770

Clark IA, Budd AC, Hsue G, Haymore BR, Joyce AJ, Thorner R, Krause PJ. Absence of erythrocyte sequestration in a case of babesiosis in a splenectomized human patient. Malar J. 2006 Aug 4;5:69. PMID:16887045

Conrad PA, Kjemtrup AM, Carreno RA, Thomford J, Wainwright K, Eberhard M, Quick R, Telford SR 3rd, Herwaldt BL. Description of Babesia duncani n.sp. (Apicomplexa: Babesiidae) from humans and its differentiation from other piroplasms. Int J Parasitol. 2006 Jun;36(7):779-89. Epub 2006 May 4. PMID:16725142

Corpelet C, Vacher P, Coudore F, Laurichesse H, Conort N, Souweine B. Role of quinine in life-threatening Babesia divergens infection successfully treated with clindamycin. Eur J Clin Microbiol Infect Dis. 2005 Jan;24(1):74-5. PMID:15616840

Cunha BA, Cohen YZ, McDermott B. Fever of unknown origin (FUO) due to babesiosis in a immunocompetent host. Heart Lung. 2008 Nov-Dec;37(6):481-4. Epub 2008 Sep 30. PMID:18992633

Cunha BA, Nausheen S, Szalda D. Pulmonary complications of babesiosis: case report and literature review. Eur J Clin Microbiol Infect Dis. 2007 Jul;26(7):505-8. PMID:17558489

Dantas-Torres F, Figueredo LA. Canine babesiosis: a Brazilian perspective. Vet Parasitol. 2006 Nov 5;141(3-4):197-203. Epub 2006 Sep 8. PMID:16962707

Dantrakool A, Somboon P, Hashimoto T, Saito-Ito A. Identification of a new type of Babesia species in wild rats (Bandicota indica) in Chiang Mai Province, Thailand. J Clin Microbiol. 2004 Feb;42(2):850-4. PMID:14766871

Delbecq S, Precigout E, Schetters T, Gorenflot A. Babesia divergens: cloning of a Ran binding protein 1 homologue. Vet Parasitol. 2003 Jul 29;115(3):205-11. PMID:12935735

Dobroszycki J, Herwaldt BL, Boctor F, Miller JR, Linden J, Eberhard ML, Yoon JJ, Ali NM, Tanowitz HB, Graham F, Weiss LM, Wittner M. A cluster of transfusion-associated babesiosis cases traced to a single asymptomatic donor. JAMA. 1999 Mar 10;281(10):927-30. PMID:10078490

Dodd JD, Aquino SL, Sharma A. Babesiosis: CT and hematologic findings. J Thorac Imaging. 2007 Aug;22(3):271-3. PMID:17721341

Dorman SE, Cannon ME, Telford SR 3rd, Frank KM, Churchill WH. Fulminant babesiosis treated with clindamycin, quinine, and whole-blood exchange transfusion. Transfusion. 2000 Mar;40(3):375-80. PMID:10738042

Duh D, Jelovsek M, Avsic-Zupanc T. Evaluation of an indirect fluorescence immunoassay for the detection of serum antibodies against Babesia divergens in humans. Parasitology. 2007 Feb;134(Pt 2):179-85. Epub 2006 Oct 11. PMID:17032478

Dvoraková HM, Dvorácková M. [Babesiosis, a little known zoonosis]. [Article in Czech]. Epidemiol Mikrobiol Imunol. 2007 Nov;56(4):176-80. PMID:18072299

El-Bahnasawy MM, Morsy TA. Egyptian human babesiosis and general review. J Egypt Soc Parasitol. 2008 Apr;38(1):265-72. PMID:19143136

Eskow ES, Krause PJ, Spielman A, Freeman K, Aslanzadeh J. Southern extension of the range of human babesiosis in the eastern United States. J Clin Microbiol. 1999 Jun;37(6):2051-2. PMID:10325378

Florescu D, Sordillo PP, Glyptis A, Zlatanic E, Smith B, Polsky B, Sordillo E. Splenic infarction in human babesiosis: two cases and discussion. Clin Infect Dis. 2008 Jan 1;46(1):e8-11. PMID:18171204

Foppa IM, Krause PJ, Spielman A, Goethert H, Gern L, Brand B, Telford SR 3rd. Entomologic and serologic evidence of zoonotic transmission of Babesia microti, eastern Switzerland. Emerg Infect Dis. 2002 Jul;8(7):722-6. PMID:12095442

Fox LM, Wingerter S, Ahmed A, Arnold A, Chou J, Rhein L, Levy O. Neonatal babesiosis: case report and review of the literature. Pediatr Infect Dis J. 2006 Feb;25(2):169-73. PMID:16462298

Froberg MK, Dannen D, Bakken JS. Babesiosis and HIV. Lancet. 2004 Feb 28;363(9410):704. PMID:15001329

Froberg MK, Dannen D, Bernier N, Shieh WJ, Guarner J, Zaki S. Case report: spontaneous splenic rupture during acute parasitemia of Babesia microti. Ann Clin Lab Sci. 2008 Autumn;38(4):390-2. PMID:18988934

Gallagher LG, Chau S, Owaisi AS, Konczyk M, Bishop HS, Arguin PM, Trenholme GM. An 84-year-old woman with fever and dark urine. Clin Infect Dis. 2009 Jul 15;49(2):278, 310-1. PMID:19538064

Gary AT, Webb JA, Hegarty BC, Breitschwerdt EB. The low seroprevalence of tick-transmitted agents of disease in dogs from southern Ontario and Quebec. Can Vet J. 2006 Dec;47(12):1194-200. PMID:17217089

Gern L, Lienhard R, Péter O. [Diseases and pathogenic agents transmitted by ticks in Switzerland].[Article in French]. Rev Med Suisse. 2010 Oct 13;6(266):1906-9. PMID:21089555

Goethert HK, Telford SR 3rd. Enzootic transmission of Babesia divergens among cottontail rabbits on Nantucket Island, Massachusetts. Am J Trop Med Hyg. 2003 Nov;69(5):455-60. PMID:14695079

Goo YK, Terkawi MA, Jia H, Aboge GO, Ooka H, Nelson B, Kim S, Sunaga F, Namikawa K, Igarashi I, Nishikawa Y, Xuan X. Artesunate, a potential drug for treatment of Babesia infection. Parasitol Int. 2010 Sep;59(3):481-6. Epub 2010 Jun 9. PMID:20541037

Guan G, Chauvin A, Yin H, Luo J, Moreau E. Course of infection by Babesia sp. BQ1 (Lintan) and B. divergens in sheep depends on the production of IFNgamma and IL10. Parasite Immunol. 2010 Feb;32(2):143-52. PMID:20070828

Gubernot DM, Lucey CT, Lee KC, Conley GB, Holness LG, Wise RP. Babesia infection through blood transfusions: reports received by the US Food and Drug Administration, 1997-2007. Clin Infect Dis. 2009 Jan 1;48(1):25-30. PMID:19035776

Gutman JD, Kotton CN, Kratz A. Case records of the Massachusetts General Hospital. Weekly clinicopathological exercises. Case 29-2003. A 60-year-old man with fever, rigors, and sweats. N Engl J Med. 2003 Sep 18;349(12):1168-75. PMID:13679532

Hamer SA, Tsao JI, Walker ED, Mansfield LS, Foster ES, Hickling GJ. Use of tick surveys and serosurveys to evaluate pet dogs as a sentinel species for emerging Lyme disease. Am J Vet Res. 2009 Jan;70(1):49-56. PMID:19119948

Han JI, Lee SJ, Jang HJ, Na KJ. Asymptomatic Babesia microti-like parasite infection in wild raccoon dogs (Nyctereutes procyonoides) in South Korea. J Wildl Dis. 2010 Apr;46(2):632-5. PMID:20688664

Harvey WT, Martz D. Motor neuron disease recovery associated with IV ceftriaxone and anti-Babesia therapy. Acta Neurol Scand. 2007 Feb;115(2):129-31. PMID:17212618

Häselbarth K, Tenter AM, Brade V, Krieger G, Hunfeld KP. First case of human babesiosis in Germany - Clinical presentation and molecular characterisation of the pathogen. Int J Med Microbiol. 2007 Jun;297(3):197-204. Epub 2007 Mar 12. PMID:17350888

Hatcher JC, Greenberg PD, Antique J, Jimenez-Lucho VE. Severe babesiosis in Long Island: review of 34 cases and their complications. Clin Infect Dis. 2001 Apr 15;32(8):1117-25. Epub 2001 Mar 26. PMID:11283800

Hemmer RM, Wozniak EJ, Lowenstine LJ, Plopper CG, Wong V, Conrad PA. Endothelial cell changes are associated with pulmonary edema and respiratory distress in mice infected with the WA1 human Babesia parasite. J Parasitol. 1999 Jun;85(3):479-89. PMID:10386441

Herman JH, Ayache S, Olkowska D. Autoimmunity in transfusion babesiosis: a spectrum of clinical presentations. J Clin Apher. 2010;25(6):358-61. Epub 2010 Sep 7. PMID:20824620

Hermanowska-Szpakowicz T, Skotarczak B, Kondrusik M, Rymaszewska A, Sawczuk M, Maciejewska A, Adamska M, Pancewicz S, Zajkowska J. Detecting DNAs of Anaplasma phagocytophilum and Babesia in the blood of patients suspected of Lyme disease. Ann Agric Environ Med. 2004;11(2):351-4. PMID:15627349

Herwaldt BL, Cacciò S, Gherlinzoni F, Aspöck H, Slemenda SB, Piccaluga P, Martinelli G, Edelhofer R, Hollenstein U, Poletti G, Pampiglione S, Löschenberger , Tura S, Pieniazek NJ. Molecular characterization of a non-Babesia divergens organism causing zoonotic babesiosis in Europe. Emerg Infect Dis. 2003 Aug;9(8):942-8. PMID:12967491

Herwaldt BL, McGovern PC, Gerwel MP, Easton RM, MacGregor RR. Endemic babesiosis in another eastern state: New Jersey. Emerg Infect Dis. 2003 Feb;9(2):184-8. PMID:12603988

Herwaldt BL, Neitzel DF, Gorlin JB, Jensen KA, Perry EH, Peglow WR, Slemenda SB,

Won KY, Nace EK, Pieniazek NJ, Wilson M. Transmission of Babesia microti in Minnesota through four blood donations from the same donor over a 6-month period. Transfusion. 2002 Sep;42(9):1154-8. PMID:12430672

Heyman P, Cochez C, Hofhuis A, van der Giessen J, Sprong H, Porter SR, Losson B, Saegerman C, Donoso-Mantke O, Niedrig M, Papa A. A clear and present danger: tick-borne diseases in Europe. Expert Rev Anti Infect Ther. 2010 Jan;8(1):33-50. PMID:20014900

Hildebrandt A, Hunfeld KP, Baier M, Krumbholz A, Sachse S, Lorenzen T, Kiehntopf M, Fricke HJ, Straube E. First confirmed autochthonous case of human Babesia microti infection in Europe. Eur J Clin Microbiol Infect Dis. 2007 Aug;26(8):595-601. PMID:17587072

Hilton E, DeVoti J, Benach JL, Halluska ML, White DJ, Paxton H, Dumler JS. Seroprevalence and seroconversion for tick-borne diseases in a high-risk population in the northeast United States. Am J Med. 1999 Apr;106(4):404-9. PMID:10225242

Hohenschild S. [Babesiosis--a dangerous infection for splenectomized children and adults].[Article in German]. Klin Padiatr. 1999 May-Jun;211(3):137-40. PMID:10412122

Holman PJ, Spencer AM, Droleskey RE, Goethert HK, Telford
SR 3rd. In vitro cultivation of a zoonotic Babesia sp. isolated from
eastern cottontail rabbits (Sylvilagus floridanus) on Nantucket
Island, Massachusetts. J Clin Microbiol. 2005 Aug;43(8):3995-4001.
PMID:16081941

Holman PJ, Spencer AM, Telford SR 3rd, Goethert HK, Allen AJ,
Knowles DP, Goff WL. Comparative infectivity of Babesia divergens
and a zoonotic Babesia divergens-like parasite in cattle. Am J Trop
Med Hyg. 2005 Nov;73(5):865-70. PMID:16282295

Homer MJ, Aguilar-Delfin I, Telford SR 3rd, Krause PJ, Persing
DH. Babesiosis. Clin Microbiol Rev. 2000 Jul;13(3):451-69.
PMID:10885987

Homer MJ, Lodes MJ, Reynolds LD, Zhang Y, Douglass JF, McNeill
PD, Houghton RL, Persing DH. Identification and characterization
of putative secreted antigens from Babesia microti. J Clin Microbiol.
2003 Feb;41(2):723-9. PMID:12574273

Houghton RL, Homer MJ, Reynolds LD, Sleath PR, Lodes MJ,
Berardi V, Leiby DA, Persing DH. Identification of Babesia
microti-specific immunodominant epitopes and development of a
peptide EIA for detection of antibodies in serum. Transfusion. 2002
Nov;42(11):1488-96. PMID:12421223

Hunfeld KP, Allwinn R, Peters S, Kraiczy P, Brade V. Serologic
evidence for tick-borne pathogens other than Borrelia burgdorferi
(TOBB) in Lyme borreliosis patients from midwestern Germany. Wien
Klin Wochenschr. 1998 Dec 23;110(24):901-8. PMID:10048174

Hunfeld KP, Brade V. Zoonotic Babesia: possibly emerging pathogens
to be considered for tick-infested humans in Central Europe. Int J Med
Microbiol. 2004 Apr;293 Suppl 37:93-103. PMID:15146990

Hunfeld KP, Hildebrandt A, Gray JS. Babesiosis: recent insights into
an ancient disease. Int J Parasitol. 2008 Sep;38(11):1219-37. Epub
2008 Mar 20. PMID:18440005

Hunfeld KP, Lambert A, Kampen H, Albert S, Epe C, Brade V, Tenter AM. Seroprevalence of Babesia infections in humans exposed to ticks in Midwestern Germany. J Clin Microbiol. 2002 Jul;40(7):2431-6. PMID:12089258

Hutchings CL, Li A, Fernandez KM, Fletcher T, Jackson LA, Molloy JB, Jorgensen WK, Lim CT, Cooke BM. New insights into the altered adhesive and mechanical properties of red blood cells parasitized by Babesia bovis. Mol Microbiol. 2007 Aug;65(4):1092-105. Epub 2007 Jul 19. PMID:17640278

Jackson LA, Waldron SJ, Weier HM, Nicoll CL, Cooke BM. Babesia bovis: culture of laboratory-adapted parasite lines and clinical isolates in a chemically defined medium. Exp Parasitol. 2001 Nov;99(3):168-74. PMID:11846527

Jahangir A, Kolbert C, Edwards W, Mitchell P, Dumler JS, Persing DH. Fatal pancarditis associated with human granulocytic Ehrlichiosis in a 44-year-old man. Clin Infect Dis. 1998 Dec;27(6):1424-7. PMID:9868655

Jeneby MM, Ngeiywa M, Yole DS, Mwenda JM, Suleman MA, Carlson HE. Enzootic simian piroplasm (Entopolypoides macaci) in wild-caught Kenyan non-human primates. J Med Primatol. 2008 Dec;37(6):329-36. Epub 2008 May 27. PMID:18507704

Kain KC, Jassoum SB, Fong IW, Hannach B. Transfusion-transmitted babesiosis in Ontario: first reported case in Canada. CMAJ. 2001 Jun 12;164(12):1721-3. PMID:11450217

Kim JY, Cho SH, Joo HN, Tsuji M, Cho SR, Park IJ, Chung GT, Ju JW, Cheun HI, Lee

HW, Lee YH, Kim TS. First case of human babesiosis in Korea: detection and characterization of a novel type of Babesia sp. (KO1) similar to ovine babesia. J Clin Microbiol. 2007 Jun;45(6):2084-7. Epub 2007 Mar 28. PMID:17392446

Kjemtrup AM, Conrad PA. A review of the small canine piroplasms from California: Babesia conradae in the literature. Vet Parasitol. 2006 May 31;138(1-2):112-7. Epub 2006 Mar 7. PMID:16522352

Kjemtrup AM, Wainwright K, Miller M, Penzhorn BL, Carreno RA. Babesia conradae, sp. Nov., a small canine Babesia identified in California. Vet Parasitol. 2006 May 31;138(1-2):103-11. Epub 2006 Mar 9. PMID:16524663

Kolören Z, Avşar C, Şekeroğlu ZA. [Diagnosis of protozoa by loop-mediated isothermal amplification: (LAMP)].[Article in Turkish]. Turkiye Parazitol Derg. 2010;34(4):207-11. PMID:21391196

Köster LS, Van Schoor M, Goddard A, Thompson PN, Matjila PT, Kjelgaard-Hansen M. C-reactive protein in canine babesiosis caused by Babesia rossi and its association with outcome. J S Afr Vet Assoc. 2009 Jun;80(2):87-91. PMID:19831269

Krause PJ. Babesiosis. Med Clin North Am. 2002 Mar;86(2):361-73. PMID:11982307

Krause PJ. Babesiosis diagnosis and treatment. Vector Borne Zoonotic Dis. 2003 Spring;3(1):45-51. PMID:12804380

Kumar S, Kumar R, Sugimoto C. A perspective on Theileria equi infections in donkeys. Jpn J Vet Res. 2009 Feb;56(4):171-80. PMID:19358444

Kuwayama DP, Briones RJ. Spontaneous splenic rupture caused by Babesia microti infection. Clin Infect Dis. 2008 May 1;46(9):e92-5. PMID:18419430

Lantos PM, Krause PJ. Babesiosis: similar to malaria but different. Pediatr Ann. 2002 Mar;31(3):192-7. PMID:11905293

Lee BP. Apnea, bradycardia and thrombocytopenia in a premature infant. Pediatr Infect Dis J. 2001 Aug;20(8):816, 820-2. PMID:11734753

Lee S, Carson K, Rice-Ficht A, Good T. Small heat shock proteins differentially affect Abeta aggregation and toxicity. Biochem Biophys Res Commun. 2006 Aug 25;347(2):527-33. Epub 2006 Jun 30. PMID:16828710

Leiby DA, Chung AP, Cable RG, Trouern-Trend J, McCullough J, Homer MJ, Reynolds LD, Houghton RL, Lodes MJ, Persing DH. Relationship between tick bites and the seroprevalence of Babesia microti and Anaplasma phagocytophila (previously Ehrlichia sp.) in blood donors. Transfusion. 2002 Dec;42(12):1585-91. PMID:12473139

Leiby DA, Chung AP, Gill JE, Houghton RL, Persing DH, Badon S, Cable RG. Demonstrable parasitemia among Connecticut blood donors with antibodies to Babesia microti. Transfusion. 2005 Nov;45(11):1804-10. PMID:16271108

Leiby DA, Gill JE. Transfusion-transmitted tick-borne infections: a cornucopia of threats. Transfus Med Rev. 2004 Oct;18(4):293-306. PMID:15497129

Leisewitz AL, Jacobson LS, de Morais HS, Reyers F. The mixed acid-base disturbances of severe canine babesiosis. J Vet Intern Med. 2001 Sep-Oct;15(5):445-52. PMID:11596731

Littman MP. Canine borreliosis. Vet Clin North Am Small Anim Pract. 2003 Jul;33(4):827-62. PMID:12910746

Loa CC, Adelson ME, Mordechai E, Raphaelli I, Tilton RC. Serological diagnosis of human babesiosis by IgG enzyme-linked immunosorbent assay. Curr Microbiol. 2004 Dec;49(6):385-9. PMID:15696612

Lodes MJ, Dillon DC, Houghton RL, Skeiky YA. Expression cloning. Methods Mol Med. 2004;94:91-106. PMID:14959824

Lodes MJ, Houghton RL, Bruinsma ES, Mohamath R, Reynolds LD, Benson DR, Krause PJ, Reed SG, Persing DH. Serological expression cloning of novel immunoreactive antigens of Babesia microti. Infect Immun. 2000 May;68(5):2783-90. PMID:10768973

Luo Y, Jia H, Terkawi MA, Goo YK, Kawano S, Ooka H, Li Y, Yu L, Cao S, Yamagishi J, Fujisaki K, Nishikawa Y, Saito-Ito A, Igarashi I, Xuan X. Identification and characterization of a novel secreted antigen 1 of Babesia microti and evaluation of its potential use in enzyme-linked immunosorbent assay and immunochromatographic test. Parasitol Int. 2011 Jun;60(2):119-25. Epub 2010 Nov 8. PMID:21070864

Lux JZ, Weiss D, Linden JV, Kessler D, Herwaldt BL, Wong SJ, Keithly J, Della-Latta P, Scully BE. Transfusion-associated babesiosis after heart transplant. Emerg Infect Dis. 2003 Jan;9(1):116-9. PMID:12533293

Marathe A, Tripathi J, Handa V, Date V. Human babesiosis--a case report. Indian J Med Microbiol. 2005 Oct;23(4):267-9. PMID:16327127

Marco I, Velarde R, Castellà J, Ferrer D, Lavín S. Presumptive Babesia ovis infection in a spanish ibex (Capra pyrenaica). Vet Parasitol. 2000 Jan;87(2-3):217-21. PMID:10622613

Marcu CB, Caracciolo E, Libertin C, Donohue T. Fulminant babesiosis manifested soon after coronary bypass surgery. Conn Med. 2005 Feb;69(2):67-8. PMID:15779600

Martinot M, Zadeh MM, Hansmann Y, Grawey I, Christmann D, Aguillon S, Jouglin M, Chauvin A, De Briel D. Babesiosis in immunocompetent patients, Europe. Emerg Infect Dis. 2011 Jan;17(1):114-6. PMID:21192869

Matsui T, Inoue R, Kajimoto K, Tamekane A, Okamura A, Katayama Y, Shimoyama M, Chihara K, Saito-Ito A, Tsuji M. [First documentation of transfusion-associated babesiosis in Japan]. [Article in Japanese]. Rinsho Ketsueki. 2000 Aug;41(8):628-34. PMID:11020989

Matthews J, Rattigan E, Yee H. Case 29-2003: a 60-year-old man with fever, rigors, and sweats. N Engl J Med. 2003 Dec 18;349(25):2467; author reply 2467. PMID:14681519

Mbati PA, Hlatshwayo M, Mtshali MS, Mogaswane KR, De Waal TD, Dipeolu OO. Ticks and tick-borne diseases of livestock belonging to resource-poor farmers in the eastern Free State of South Africa. Exp Appl Acarol. 2002;28(1-4):217-24. PMID:14570134

Meer-Scherrer L, Adelson M, Mordechai E, Lottaz B, Tilton R. Babesia microti infection in Europe. Curr Microbiol. 2004 Jun;48(6):435-7. PMID:15170239

Meister J. Human babesiosis: a case study. Clin Excell Nurse Pract. 1999 Jul;3(4):214-6. PMID:10711060

Mitrović S, Kranjcić-Zec I, Arsić-Arsenijević V, Dzamić A, Radonjić I. [Human babesiosis--recent discoveries].[Article in Serbian]. Med Pregl. 2004 Jul-Aug;57(7-8):349-53. PMID:15626291

Montero E, Rodriguez M, Oksov Y, Lobo CA. Babesia divergens apical membrane antigen 1 and its interaction with the human red blood cell. Infect Immun. 2009 Nov;77(11):4783-93. Epub 2009 Aug 31. PMID:19720759

Moreno Giménez JC, Jiménez Puya R, Galán Gutiérrez M, Ortega Salas R, Dueñas Jurado JM. Erythema figuratum in septic babesiosis. J Eur Acad Dermatol Venereol. 2006 Jul;20(6):726-8. PMID:16836504

Mylonakis E. When to suspect and how to monitor babesiosis. Am Fam Physician. 2001 May 15;63(10):1969-74. PMID:11388711

Nagao E, Arie T, Dorward DW, Fairhurst RM, Dvorak JA. The avian malaria parasite Plasmodium gallinaceum causes marked structural changes on the surface of its host erythrocyte. J Struct Biol. 2008 Jun;162(3):460-7. Epub 2008 Mar 21. PMID:18442920

Narasimhan S, Montgomery RR, DePonte K, Tschudi C, Marcantonio N, Anderson JF, Sauer JR, Cappello M, Kantor FS, Fikrig E. Disruption of Ixodes scapularis anticoagulation by using RNA interference. Proc Natl Acad Sci U S A. 2004 Feb 3;101(5):1141-6. Epub 2004 Jan 26. PMID:14745044

Ngo V, Civen R. Babesiosis acquired through blood transfusion, California, USA. Emerg Infect Dis. 2009 May;15(5):785-7. PMID:19402969

Nicholson GT, Walsh CA, Madan RP. Transfusion-associated babesiosis in a 7-month-old infant after bidirectional Glenn procedure. Congenit Heart Dis. 2010 Nov-Dec;5(6):607-13. PMID:21106022

Nishisaka M, Yokoyama N, Xuan X, Inoue N, Nagasawa H, Fujisaki K, Mikami T, Igarashi I. Characterisation of the gene encoding a protective antigen from Babesia microti identified it as eta subunit of chaperonin containing T-complex protein 1. Int J Parasitol. 2001 Dec;31(14):1673-9. PMID:11730795

Nohýnková E, Kubek J, Měst'ánková O, Chalupa P, Hubálek Z. [A case of Babesia microti imported into the Czech Republic from the USA].[Article in Czech]. Cas Lek Cesk. 2003;142(6):377-81. PMID:12924039

Oleson CV, Sivalingam JJ, O'Neill BJ, Staas WE Jr. Transverse myelitis secondary to coexistent Lyme disease and babesiosis. J Spinal Cord Med. 2003 Summer;26(2):168-71. PMID:12828297

Oliveira TM, Furuta PI, de Carvalho D, Machado RZ. A study of cross-reactivity in serum samples from dogs positive for Leishmania sp., Babesia canis and Ehrlichia canis in enzyme-linked immunosorbent assay and indirect fluorescent antibody test. Rev Bras Parasitol Vet. 2008 Jan-Mar;17(1):7-11. PMID:18554433

Ooka H, Terkawi MA, Goo YK, Luo Y, Li Y, Yamagishi J, Nishikawa Y, Igarashi I, Xuan X. Babesia microti: molecular and antigenic characterizations of a novel 94-kDa protein (BmP94). Exp Parasitol. 2011 Jan;127(1):287-93. Epub 2010 Jun 25. PMID:20599995

Pancewicz S, Moniuszko A, Bieniarz E, Puciło K, Grygorczuk S, Zajkowska J, Czupryna P, Kondrusik M, Swierzbińska-Pijanowska R. Anti-Babesia microti antibodies in foresters highly exposed to tick bites in Poland. Scand J Infect Dis. 2011 Mar;43(3):197-201. Epub 2010 Dec 9. PMID:21142620

Pantanowitz L, Aufranc S 3rd, Monahan-Earley R, Dvorak A, Telford SR 3rd. Transfusion medicine illustrated. Morphologic hallmarks of Babesia. Transfusion. 2002 Nov;42(11):1389. PMID:12421208

Pendse S, Bilyk JR, Lee MS. The ticking time bomb. Surv Ophthalmol. 2006 May-Jun;51(3):274-9. PMID:16644367

Perdrizet GA, Olson NH, Krause PJ, Banever GT, Spielman A, Cable RG. Babesiosis in a renal transplant recipient acquired through blood transfusion. Transplantation. 2000 Jul 15;70(1):205-8. PMID:10919602

Permin A, Yelifari L, Bloch P, Steenhard N, Hansen NP, Nansen P. Parasites in cross-bred pigs in the Upper East region of Ghana. Vet Parasitol. 1999 Nov;87(1):63-71. PMID:10628701

Precigout E, Delbecq S, Vallet A, Carcy B, Camillieri S, Hadj-Kaddour K, Kleuskens J, Schetters T, Gorenflot A. Association between sequence polymorphism in an epitope of Babesia divergens Bd37 exoantigen and protection induced by passive transfer. Int J Parasitol. 2004 Apr;34(5):585-93. PMID:15064123

Prince HE, Lapé-Nixon M, Patel H, Yeh C. Comparison of the Babesia duncani (WA1) IgG detection rates among clinical sera submitted to a reference laboratory for WA1 IgG testing and blood donor specimens from diverse geographic areas of the United States. Clin Vaccine Immunol. 2010 Nov;17(11):1729-33. Epub 2010 Sep 22. PMID:20861326

Qi C, Zhou D, Liu J, Cheng Z, Zhang L, Wang L, Wang Z, Yang D, Wang S, Chai T. Detection of Babesia divergens using molecular methods in anemic patients in Shandong Province, China. Parasitol Res. 2011 Jul;109(1):241-5. Epub 2011 Apr 19. PMID:21503639

Quintão-Silva MG, Melo MN, Ribeiro MF. Comparison of duplex PCR and microscopic techniques for the identification of Babesia bigemina and Babesia bovis in engorged female ticks of Boophilus microplus. Zoonoses Public Health. 2007;54(3-4):147-51. PMID:17456146

Raju M, Salazar JC, Leopold H, Krause PJ. Atovaquone and azithromycin treatment for babesiosis in an infant. Pediatr Infect Dis J. 2007 Feb;26(2):181-3. PMID:17259886

Ramharter M, Walochnik J, Lagler H, Winkler S, Wernsdorfer WH, Stoiser B, Graninger W. Clinical and molecular characterization of a near fatal case of human babesiosis in Austria. J Travel Med. 2010 Nov-Dec;17(6):416-8. PMID:21050324

Rech A, Bittar CM, de Castro CG, Azevedo KR, dos Santos RP, Machado AR, Schwartsmann G, Goldani L, Brunetto AL. Asymptomatic babesiosis in a child with hepatoblastoma. J Pediatr Hematol Oncol. 2004 Mar;26(3):213. PMID:15125618

Reis C, Cote M, Paul RE, Bonnet S. Questing ticks in suburban forest are infected by at least six tick-borne pathogens. Vector Borne Zoonotic Dis. 2011 Jul;11(7):907-16. Epub 2010 Dec 15. PMID:21158500

Reis SP, Maddineni S, Rozenblit G, Allen D. Spontaneous splenic rupture secondary to Babesia microti infection: treatment with splenic artery embolization. J Vasc Interv Radiol. 2011 May;22(5):732-4. PMID:21514529

Ríos L, Alvarez G, Blair S. Serological and parasitological study and report of the first case of human babesiosis in Colombia. Rev Soc Bras Med Trop. 2003 Jul-Aug;36(4):493-8. Epub 2003 Aug 13. PMID:12937727

Rosenblatt JE. Laboratory diagnosis of infections due to blood and tissue parasites. Clin Infect Dis. 2009 Oct 1;49(7):1103-8. PMID:19691431

Ryan R, Krause PJ, Radolf J, Freeman K, Spielman A, Lenz R, Levin A. Diagnosis of babesiosis using an immunoblot serologic test. Clin Diagn Lab Immunol. 2001 Nov;8(6):1177-80. PMID:11687460

Saito-Ito A, Dantrakool A, Kawai A, Yano Y, Takada N. [Babesiosis]. [Article in Japanese]. Nihon Rinsho. 2003 Feb;61 Suppl 2:623-8. PMID:12722292

Saito-Ito A, Tsuji M, Wei Q, He S, Matsui T, Kohsaki M, Arai S, Kamiyama T, Hioki K, Ishihara C. Transfusion-acquired, autochthonous human babesiosis in Japan: isolation of Babesia microti-like parasites with hu-RBC-SCID mice. J Clin Microbiol. 2000 Dec;38(12):4511-6. PMID:11101588

Sambri V, Marangoni A, Storni E, Cavrini F, Moroni A, Sparacino M, Cevenini R. [Tick borne zoonosis: selected clinical and diagnostic aspects].[Article in Italian]. Parassitologia. 2004 Jun;46(1-2):109-13. PMID:15305697

Schaller JL, Burkland GA, Langhoff PJ. Are various Babesia species a missed cause for hypereosinophilia? A follow-up on the first reported case of imatinib mesylate for idiopathic hypereosinophilia. MedGenMed. 2007 Feb 27;9(1):38. PMID:17435644

Schetters TP, Eling WM. Can Babesia infections be used as a model for cerebral malaria? Parasitol Today. 1999 Dec;15(12):492-7. PMID:10557150

Schoeler GB, Manweiler SA, Wikel SK. Ixodes scapularis: effects of repeated infestations with pathogen-free nymphs on macrophage and T lymphocyte cytokine responses of BALB/c and C3H/HeN mice. Exp Parasitol. 1999 Aug;92(4):239-48. PMID:10425152

Schoeman JP. Canine babesiosis. Onderstepoort J Vet Res. 2009 Mar;76(1):59-66. PMID:19967929

Schoeman JP, Herrtage ME. Adrenal response to the low dose ACTH stimulation test and the cortisol-to-adrenocorticotrophic hormone ratio in canine babesiosis. Vet Parasitol. 2008 Jul 4;154(3-4):205-13. Epub 2008 Apr 7. PMID:18468798

Semel ME, Tavakkolizadeh A, Gates JD. Babesiosis in the immediate postoperative period after splenectomy for trauma. Surg Infect (Larchmt). 2009 Dec;10(6):553-6. PMID:19622029

Sethi S, Alcid D, Kesarwala H, Tolan RW Jr. Probable congenital babesiosis in infant, new jersey, USA. Emerg Infect Dis. 2009 May;15(5):788-91. PMID:19402971

Setty S, Khalil Z, Schori P, Azar M, Ferrieri P. Babesiosis. Two atypical cases from Minnesota and a review. Am J Clin Pathol. 2003 Oct;120(4):554-9. PMID:14560566

Sherr VT. Human babesiosis--an unrecorded reality. Absence of formal registry undermines its detection, diagnosis and treatment, suggesting need for immediate mandatory reporting. Med Hypotheses. 2004;63(4):609-15. PMID:15325004

Shoemaker RC, Hudnell HK, House DE, Van Kempen A, Pakes GE; COL40155 Study Team. Atovaquone plus cholestyramine in patients coinfected with Babesia microti and Borrelia burgdorferi refractory to other treatment. Adv Ther. 2006 Jan-Feb;23(1):1-11. PMID:16644602

Skotarczak B. [Babesiosis of human and domestic dog; ethiology, pathogenesis, diagnostics].[Article in Polish]. Wiad Parazytol. 2007;53(4):271-80. PMID:18441872

Skotarczak B, Cichocka A. Isolation and amplification by polymerase chain reaction DNA of Babesia microti and Babesia divergens in ticks in Poland. Ann Agric Environ Med. 2001;8(2):187-9. PMID:11748876

Skotarczak B, Sawczuk M. [Occurrence of Babesia microti in ticks Ixodes ricinus on selected areas of western Pomerania].[Article in Polish]. Wiad Parazytol. 2003;49(3):273-80. PMID:16889031

Sréter T, Sréterné Lancz Z, Széll Z, Egyed L. [Rickettsia helvetica: an emerging tick-borne pathogen in Hungary and Europe]. [Article in Hungarian]. Orv Hetil. 2005 Dec 11;146(50):2547-52. PMID:16440500

Sréter T, Kálmán D, Sréterné Lancz Z, Széll Z, Egyed L. [Babesia microti and Anaplasma phagocytophilum: two emerging zoonotic pathogens in Europe and Hungary].[Article in Hungarian]. Orv Hetil. 2005 Mar 27;146(13):595-600. PMID:15856623

Stańczak J, Myjak P, Bajer A, Siński E, Wedrychowicz H, Majewska AC, Gołab E, Budak A. [Usefulness of the molecular techniques for detecting and/or identifing of parasites and fungi in humans and animals or pathogens transmitted by ticks. Part III].[Article in Polish]. Wiad Parazytol. 2001;47(3):465-75. PMID:16894762

Stricker RB. Counterpoint: long-term antibiotic therapy improves persistent symptoms associated with lyme disease. Clin Infect Dis. 2007 Jul 15;45(2):149-57. Epub 2007 Jun 5. PMID:17578772

Stricker RB, Lautin A, Burrascano JJ. Lyme disease: point/ counterpoint. Expert Rev Anti Infect Ther. 2005 Apr;3(2):155-65. PMID:15918774

Taiwo B, Lee C, Venkat D, Tambar S, Sutton SH. Can tumor necrosis factor alpha blockade predispose to severe babesiosis? Arthritis Rheum. 2007 Feb 15;57(1):179-81. PMID:17266091

Tajima T, Zhi N, Lin Q, Rikihisa Y, Horowitz HW, Ralfalli J, Wormser GP, Hechemy KE. Comparison of two recombinant major outer membrane proteins of the human granulocytic ehrlichiosis agent for use in an enzyme-linked immunosorbent assay. Clin Diagn Lab Immunol. 2000 Jul;7(4):652-7. PMID:10882667

Talour K, Karam A, Dreux N, Lemasson G, Gilbert D, Abasq C, Misery L. Incipiens linear IgA disease with IgA antibodies directed against 200-kDa epidermal antigens. Eur J Dermatol. 2011 May-Jun;21(3):411-2. PMID:21515442

Terkawi MA, Jia H, Zhou J, Lee EG, Igarashi I, Fujisaki K, Nishikawa Y, Xuan X. Babesia gibsoni ribosomal phosphoprotein P0 induces cross-protective immunity against B. microti infection in mice. Vaccine. 2007 Mar 1;25(11):2027-35. Epub 2006 Dec 8. PMID:17229504

Tonnetti L, Eder AF, Dy B, Kennedy J, Pisciotto P, Benjamin RJ, Leiby DA. Transfusion-transmitted Babesia microti identified through hemovigilance. Transfusion. 2009 Dec;49(12):2557-63. Epub 2009 Jul 16. PMID:19624607

Topolovec J, Puntarić D, Antolović-Pozgain A, Vuković D, Topolovec Z, Milas J, Drusko-Barisić V, Venus M. Serologically detected "new" tick-borne zoonoses in eastern Croatia. Croat Med J. 2003 Oct;44(5):626-9. PMID:14515426

Torina A, Caracappa S. Anaplasmosis in cattle in Italy. Vet Res Commun. 2007 Aug;31 Suppl 1:73-8. PMID:17682850

Torina A, Vicente J, Alongi A, Scimeca S, Turlá R, Nicosia S, Di Marco V, Caracappa S, de la Fuente J. Observed prevalence of tick-borne pathogens in domestic animals in Sicily, Italy during 2003-2005. Zoonoses Public Health. 2007;54(1):8-15. PMID:17359441

Torres-Vélez FJ, Nace EK, Won KY, Bartlett J, Eberhard M, Guarner J. Development of an immunohistochemical assay for the detection of babesiosis in formalin-fixed, paraffin-embedded tissue samples. Am J Clin Pathol. 2003 Dec;120(6):833-8. PMID:14671971

Tsuji N, Miyoshi T, Battsetseg B, Matsuo T, Xuan X, Fujisaki K. A cysteine protease is critical for Babesia spp. transmission in Haemaphysalis ticks. PLoS Pathog. 2008 May 16;4(5):e1000062. PMID:18483546

Tuo W, Estes DM, Brown WC. Comparative effects of interleukin-12 and interleukin-4 on cytokine responses by antigen-stimulated memory CD4+ T cells of cattle: IL-12 enhances IFN-gamma production, whereas IL-4 has marginal effects on cytokine expression. J Interferon Cytokine Res. 1999 Jul;19(7):741-9. PMID:10454344

van Duivenvoorde LM, Voorberg-van der Wel A, van der Werff NM, Braskamp G, Remarque EJ, Kondova I, Kocken CH, Thomas AW. Suppression of Plasmodium cynomolgi in rhesus macaques by coinfection with Babesia microti. Infect Immun. 2010 Mar;78(3):1032-9. Epub 2010 Jan 4. PMID:20048045

Van Solingen RM, Evans J. Lyme disease. Curr Opin Rheumatol. 2001 Jul;13(4):293-9. PMID:11555731

Vannier E, Gewurz BE, Krause PJ. Human babesiosis. Infect Dis Clin North Am. 2008 Sep;22(3):469-88, viii-ix. PMID:18755385

Vannier E, Krause PJ. Update on babesiosis. Interdiscip Perspect Infect Dis. 2009;2009:984568. Epub 2009 Aug 27. PMID:19727410

Vyas JM, Telford SR, Robbins GK. Treatment of refractory Babesia microti infection with atovaquone-proguanil in an HIV-infected patient: case report. Clin Infect Dis. 2007 Dec 15;45(12):1588-90. PMID:18190320

Wang TJ, Liang MH, Sangha O, Phillips CB, Lew RA, Wright EA, Berardi V, Fossel AH, Shadick NA. Coexposure to Borrelia burgdorferi and Babesia microti does not worsen the long-term outcome of lyme disease. Clin Infect Dis. 2000 Nov;31(5):1149-54. Epub 2000 Nov 6. PMID:11073744

Weinberg GA. Laboratory diagnosis of ehrlichiosis and babesiosis. Pediatr Infect Dis J. 2001 Apr;20(4):435-7. PMID:11332670

Weiss LM. Babesiosis in humans: a treatment review. Expert Opin Pharmacother. 2002 Aug;3(8):1109-15. PMID:12150690

Wójcik-Fatla A, Cisak E, Chmielewska-Badora J, Zwoliński J, Buczek A, Dutkiewicz

J. Prevalence of Babesia microti in Ixodes ricinus ticks from Lublin region (eastern Poland). Ann Agric Environ Med. 2006;13(2):319-22. PMID:17196008

Wong WS, Chung JY, Wong KF. Images in haematology. Human babesiosis. Br J Haematol. 2008 Feb;140(4):364. Epub 2007 Nov 27. PMID:18042268

Wormser GP, Lombardo G, Silverblatt F, El Khoury MY, Prasad A, Yelon JA, Sanda A, Karim S, Coku L, Savino JA. Babesiosis as a cause of fever in patients undergoing a splenectomy. Am Surg. 2011 Mar;77(3):345-7. PMID:21375849

Wormser GP, Prasad A, Neuhaus E, Joshi S, Nowakowski J, Nelson J, Mittleman A, Aguero-Rosenfeld M, Topal J, Krause PJ. Emergence of resistance to azithromycin-atovaquone in immunocompromised patients with Babesia microti infection. Clin Infect Dis. 2010 Feb 1;50(3):381-6. PMID:20047477

Yabsley MJ, Davidson WR, Stallknecht DE, Varela AS, Swift PK, Devos JC Jr, Dubay SA. Evidence of tick-borne organisms in mule deer (Odocoileus hemionus) from the western United States. Vector Borne Zoonotic Dis. 2005 Winter;5(4):351-62. PMID:16417431

Yabsley MJ, Romines J, Nettles VF. Detection of Babesia and Anaplasma species in rabbits from Texas and Georgia, USA. Vector Borne Zoonotic Dis. 2006 Spring;6(1):7-13. PMID:16584322

Yamasaki M, Tajima M, Yamato O, Hwang SJ, Ohta H, Maede Y. Heat shock response of Babesia gibsoni heat shock protein 70. J Parasitol. 2008 Feb;94(1):119-24. PMID:18372630

Yoshinari NH, Abrão MG, Bonoldi VL, Soares CO, Madruga CR, Scofield A, Massard CL, da Fonseca AH. Coexistence of antibodies to tick-borne agents of babesiosis and Lyme borreliosis in patients from Cotia county, State of São Paulo, Brazil. Mem Inst Oswaldo Cruz. 2003 Apr;98(3):311-8. Epub 2003 Jul 18. PMID:12886408

Yu DH, Li YH, Yoon JS, Lee JH, Lee MJ, Yu IJ, Chae JS, Park JH. Ehrlichia chaffeensis infection in dogs in South Korea. Vector Borne Zoonotic Dis. 2008 Jun;8(3):355-8. PMID:18399775

Zamoto A, Tsuji M, Kawabuchi T, Wei Q, Asakawa M, Ishihara C. U.S.-type Babesia microti isolated from small wild mammals in Eastern Hokkaido, Japan. J Vet Med Sci. 2004 Aug;66(8):919-26. PMID:15353841

Zamoto A, Tsuji M, Wei Q, Cho SH, Shin EH, Kim TS, Leonova GN, Hagiwara K, Asakawa M, Kariwa H, Takashima I, Ishihara C. Epizootiologic survey for Babesia microti among small wild mammals in northeastern Eurasia and a geographic diversity in the beta-tubulin gene sequences. J Vet Med Sci. 2004 Jul;66(7):785-92. PMID:15297749

Zhao Y, Love KR, Hall SW, Beardell FV. A fatal case of transfusion-transmitted babesiosis in the State of Delaware. Transfusion. 2009 Dec;49(12):2583-7. Epub 2009 Nov 9. PMID:19906041

Zivkovic Z, Torina A, Mitra R, Alongi A, Scimeca S, Kocan KM, Galindo RC, Almazán C, Blouin EF, Villar M, Nijhof AM, Mani R, La Barbera G, Caracappa S, Jongejan F, de la Fuente J. Subolesin expression in response to pathogen infection in ticks. BMC Immunol. 2010 Feb 19;11:7. PMID:20170494

Zobba R, Parpaglia ML, Spezzigu A, Pittau M, Alberti A. First molecular identification and phylogeny of a Babesia sp. from a symptomatic sow (Sus scrofa Linnaeus 1758). J Clin Microbiol. 2011 Jun;49(6):2321-4. Epub 2011 Apr 13. PMID:21490184

LYME DISEASE SYMPTOM CHECKLIST
James Schaller, M.D., M.A.R.

INTRODUCTION

The following checklist is not meant to be complete or authoritative. Information about Lyme disease is constantly emerging and changing. Therefore any checklist is intended for use as a starting point.   In traditional medicine, a physician performs a complete history and physical. Labs and studies **assist** in clarifying the differential diagnosis. In Lyme disease, much debate exists about laboratory kits, the alteration of kits to have fewer possible bands, and which labs are optimally sensitive and specific.   This checklist is not intended to address that issue or treatment.

Over 200 animals carry the Ixodes tick, which is the most commonly known insect spreading Lyme disease.   With so many vectors, the underlying assumption behind this checklist is that Lyme is not rare in North America, Europe, South America, Russia, Africa or Asia.

We know Lyme disease is highly under-reported.   One study showed only 1 in 40 family doctors reported it.

Immediately upon biting, the tick transmits a pain killer, anti-histamine and an anti-coagulant.   Based on animal studies, it is also possible the bulls-eye rash is less common than assumed, in part because injections of spirochete related material in laboratory animals only show a rash with the **second** injection. With this background, I would appeal, that if a young or middle aged adult experiences a bite, and has profound symptoms, is it possible this was a small number of infectious particles igniting a larger number from 2, 5 or 20 years earlier?   I am not asking for an answer, just for the possibility to be considered.

This checklist is offered with the sincere wish that others will improve on it.   It is this author's personal belief that tick and flea-borne infection medicine is as specialized as HIV and Hepatitis medical science and treatment.

Some of the checklist materials might be new to you, which underscores the need for another scale to add to the ones currently in existence. This list is based on a massive review of thousands of papers over a decade of full-time reading, 2012 science revelations, and/or massive chart reviews.   Since modern Lyme disease seems to focus on tick-borne disease and other laboratory testing, we will start with lab testing considerations.   If a lab test has a value or a percentage, the numbers chosen are intended to avoid missing those positive patients who otherwise would be overlooked.   The concern is about physicians and other healthcare workers not treating an infected patient, who over time can experience disability or even death at a frequency that is impossible to determine.

THE LYME DISEASE CHECKLIST

James Schaller, M.D., M.A.R.

(Please Check Any Symptoms That Apply)

LABORATORY TESTING — INDIRECT AND DIRECT

☐ Vitamin D level is in the lowest 20%. If you supplement, it should be in top 50%.

☐ CD57 or CD58 is in the lowest 20th percentile.

☐ Free testosterone is in 10th percentile or below.

☐ In 5% of patients the testosterone or free testosterone is over the normal range.

☐ DHEA is in lower 20%. Or rarely is it fully over the top level.

☐ Free dihydrotestosterone is in the lowest 20th percentile or well over the normal range.

☐ Epstein Barr Virus is abnormal in any measure. [This virus is believed to be positive over normal positive levels in the presence of infections or high inflammation.]

☐ On the Western Blot, IgG or IgM any *species specific* band at any blood level, e.g., 18, 21, 23, 30, 31, 34, 37, 39, 83, 93.

☐ A free T3 level under 2.8 [the normal bottom range in 1990 was 2.6; the influx of large numbers of elderly patients reset the healthy "normal" range].

☐ Positive for viruses such as CMV, HHV-6, Coxsackie B Types 1, 2, 3, 4, 5, 6, Parvo B-19 or Powassan virus

☐ Positive for Mycoplasma, e.g. mycoplasma pneumonia

☐ The patient is positive for infections other than **routine** Lyme, [that is **Borrelia burgdorferi sensu stricto,** Borrelia **afzelii** and Borrelia **garinii**]. Some of the other infections also carried by infectious ticks, fleas or other vectors include Babesia (duncani, microti or other), Anaplasma (HGA), Ehrlichia (various species/ strains), Neoehrlichia, Rocky Mountain or other Spotted Fevers, Brucellosis, Q-fever, STARI (Master's Disease), Malaria, and Bartonella [e.g., B. henselae, B. quintana, B. elizabethae and B. melophagi].   Once tests are commercially available for testing all forms of protozoa affecting humans, including FL1953, all Bartonella species, and Borrelia miyamotoi and other Lyme species, reporting should increase.

☐ IL-B is in lowest 10th percentile.

☐ IL-6 is in lowest 10th percentile.

☐ TNF-alpha is under 2, or in lowest 20th percentile.

☐ A WBC count was, or is, under 4.5.

☐ Eosinophil level in the CBC manual exam is either at 0-1 or 6-7.

☐ Total manual Eosinophil level is 140 or less.

☐ X-ray or other study shows cartilage defects in excess of injury or age median.

☐ If a full auto-immunity panel is run with at least eight different tests, two are positive; for example, you have a positive anti-gliadin and a positive thyroid peroxidase.

☐ Positive or near positive (borderline) ELISA, PCR, or a positive tissue biopsy; or a tick from your body is positive for Lyme or other tick infection

☐ Lab tests show high inflammation, e.g., a high C4a, elevated cholesterol and C-peptide.   These are never specific just for Lyme.

☐ Lab tests show a MSH level under 30 [the reference range of 0-40 is due to the increase of very sick patients tested, and 40-85 is a better reference range which was used before the flood of the sick reset the range of normal]. MSH is an anti-inflammatory hormone.

☐ VIP is under 20. This is an anti-inflammation chemical.

BODY EXAMINATION RESULTS

☐ Weight loss or gain in excess of 20 pounds in 12 weeks

☐ A round or oval rash with a dark center was or is present in a loose "bulls-eye pattern" or other size and shape rashes that have no other cause after exposure to ticks and vectors

☐ Healing is slow after scratches or surgery. For example, after a cat scratch, flea bite or tick bite the mark is still visible later.

☐ Skin on arms, hands or feet has a texture like rice paper.

☐ Clear reaction and effect is seen with antibiotic treatment. Specifically, a marked improvement or worsening of a serious medical problem or function is observed with a spirochete killing treatment, e.g., doxycycline, tetracycline, minocycline, any penicillin such as amoxicillin, azithromycin, clarithromycin or cefuroxime.

☐ Presence of skin tags, red papules of any size, excess blood vessels compared to peers, and stretch marks with color or in significant excess of peers.

☐ Moles and raised or hard plaques in excess of the few on normal skin

☐ Areas of skin with ulcerations such as those seen in syphilis, but at any location on the body

☐ Areas of clear hypo-pigmentation and hyper-pigmentation

☐ Positive ACA (Acrodermatitis chronica atrophicans) which is a sign of long term untreated Lyme disease. Some report ACA begins as a reddish-blue patch of discolored skin, often of the hands or feet. It may include the back in some patients. The lesion slowly atrophies over months to years, with many developing skin that is thin, dry, hairless, wrinkled and abnormally colored. The color of the extremities such as hands and feet can be red, dark red, brown, dark blue or purple.

Sample Neurological Exam

☐ Patient's short-term memory is poor. For example, if asked to recall these numbers—23, 5, 76, 43 and 68—the patient cannot recall them.

☐ Patient cannot reverse four numbers, so if given—18, 96, 23 and 79—the patient cannot do it.

☐ If asked to subtract 17 from 120, (college graduate), it cannot be done in a timely manner. If a high school graduate, subtract 7 from 100 and continue to subtract by 7 four times in 20 seconds.

☐ Light headedness upon standing quickly in excess of peers, and with no clear cause

☐ Dizziness unrelated to position

☐ Dizziness made worse by Lyme killing antibiotics

☐ Trouble doing a nine step **heel to toe straight line walk test** with fingers slightly in pockets [The patient should not sway or need their hands pulled out to prevent a fall]. In patients with past experience in skating, skiing, dance or ballet this should be *very easy* and is rarely a challenge to such people. If it is not easy, it is suspicious medically, but not only for Lyme disease.

☐ Trouble performing a one leg lift, in which one leg is lifted 15 inches off the ground in front of you, as you count, e.g., "one Mississippi, two Mississippi, etc."

☐ Positive nystagmus [your eye jerks when you look right or left]

PATIENT'S REPORTED PHYSICAL HISTORY

Psychiatric & Neurological

☐ Mild to severe neurological disorders or psychiatric disorders

☐ A very profound neurological disease which does not clearly fit the labs, studies and course of the illness

☐ A moderate or severe medical, psychiatric or neurological illness. [Many severe disorders can be associated with spirochetes such as those causing syphilis, and some propose that Lyme is also related to a well-known serious brain disease.]

☐ Severe medical, psychiatric or neurology illness with uncommon features, such as Parkinson's disease, appearing at a young age

☐ Facial paralysis (Bell's palsy)

☐ Personality has changed negatively and significantly for no clear reason.

☐ Psychosis at any age, but especially after 40 years of age when *usually* it would have already manifested itself

☐ Severe anxiety

☐ Mania or profound rage

☐ Depression with minimal genetic risk

☐ Depression or anxiety that did not exist when you were less than 25 years of age

☐ Irritability

☐ Any one of the following: paranoia, dementia, schizophrenia, bipolar disorder, panic attacks, major depression, anorexia nervosa or obsessive-compulsive disorder

☐ Adult onset ADHD/ADD [Primary psychiatric biological ADD or ADHD is present at 7 years of age.   Adult onset is a sign of a medical condition.]

☐ Increased verbal or physical fighting with others

☐ Functioning at work or in parenting is at least 20% reduced

☐ Patience and relational skills are decreased by 20% or more

☐ A mild to profound decrease of insight, i.e., an infected patient does not see their decreased function, failed treatment or personality change

☐ A new eccentric rigidity to hearing new medical or other important information

☐ Difficulty thinking or concentrating

☐ Poor memory and reduced ability to concentrate

☐ Increasingly difficult to recall names of people or things

☐ Difficulty speaking or reading

☐ Difficulty finding the words to express what you want to say

☐ Inability to learn new information as well as in the past [receptive learning]

☐ Repeating stories or forgetting information told to close relations, such as a spouse, roommate, sibling, best friend or parent

☐ Confusion without a clear reason

☐ An addiction that results in relapse in spite of sincere, reasonable and serious efforts to stop

☐ Fatigue in excess of normal, or fatigue that is getting worse

☐ Trouble sleeping including mild to severe insomnia and disrupted sleep

☐ Sleep in excess of 9 hours a day or night, or sleeping in excess of 9 hours every day if allowed

☐ Trouble falling asleep

☐ Trouble staying asleep [Taking a 5 minute bathroom break does not count]

Major Organs

☐ Gastritis or stomach sensitivity not caused by H. Pylori

☐ Intestinal troubles that are unable to be fully managed and/or which have no clear diagnosis

☐ Nausea without a clear reason

☐ Ear problems such as pain or increased ear "pressure"

☐ *Any trouble* with the senses (vision, sound, touch, taste or smell). The use of corrective lenses or contacts does not count, unless the prescription is changed more than expected.

☐ Buzzing or ringing in ears

☐ Double vision, floaters, dry eyes, or other vision trouble

☐ Conjunctivitis (pinkeye) or occasional damage to deep tissue in the eyes

☐ Bladder dysfunction of any kind

☐ Treatment resistant interstitial cystitis

☐ Blood clots fast when you get a cut, or you have a diagnosed problem with clotting.   This may also be seen in blood draws where blood draw needle clots when blood is being removed. If on a blood thinner, blood thinness level goes up and down too much.

☐ Cardiac impairment

☐ Chest pain with all labs and studies in normal range

☐ Occasional rapid heartbeats (palpitations)

☐ Heart block/heart murmur

☐ Heart valve prolapse

☐ Shortness of breath with no clear cause on pulmonary function tests, examination, lab testing, X-rays, MRI's, etc.

☐ Air hunger or feelings of shortness of breath

Skin

☐ Numbness, tingling, burning, or shock sensations in an area of skin

☐ One or more troublesome skin sensations that move over months or years and do not always stay in one location

☐ Rash or rashes without a simple and obvious cause

☐ Rashes that persist despite treatment

☐ Eccentric itching with no clear cause

☐ Hair loss with no clear cause

Musculoskeletal

☐ Muscle pain or cramps

☐ Muscle spasms

☐ Muscle wasting without a clear cause

☐ Trouble with your jaw muscle(s) or joint insomnia (TMJ)

☐ Joint defects in one joint with no clear cause if 20 or younger

☐ Joint defects in two joints or more if 35 or younger

☐ Joint defects in three or more locations if younger than 55 with no clear trauma

☐ Swelling or pain (inflammation) in the joints [Most patients *never* have joint disease.]

☐ Joint pain that shifts location

☐ Neck stiffness

☐ Chronic arthritis with or without episodes of swelling, redness, and fluid buildup

General Medical

☐ Gaining or losing weight in a manner clearly inconsistent with diet and exercise

☐ New or more food allergies than ten years ago

☐ Feel worse after eating breads, pasta or sweets

☐ No longer tolerate or enjoy alcohol

☐ Anti-histamines are bothersome, more so than in the past.

☐ Reaction to medications is excessive (you are very "sensitive" to medications)

☐ Your response to antibiotics is significantly positive and you feel more functional, *or you have the opposite reaction* and feel worse, feeling ill, fatigued or agitated.

☐ Chronic pain in excess of what seems reasonable

☐ Nerve pain without a clear cause

☐ Sensitivity to lights, sounds, touch, smell or unusual tastes

☐ Sensitivity to cleaning chemicals, fragrances and perfumes

☐ Headaches that do not respond fully to treatment, or which are getting worse

☐ New allergies or increased allergies over those of your peers

☐ Any autoimmunity--Lyme and other tick infections, over many years, increase inflammation and decrease anti-inflammation chemicals.   We believe this leads to increased food sensitivities, increased autoimmunity and a heightened sensitivity to various chemicals and medications.

☐ Day time sweats

☐ Night time sweats

☐ Chills

☐ Flu-like symptoms

☐ Abnormal menstrual cycle

☐ Decreased or increased libido

☐ Increased motion sickness

☐ Fainting

☐ A spinning sensation or vertigo

☐ Illnesses that come and go and decrease functioning with no certain cause

☐ Serious illnesses that undermine function with no clear cause, and which affect more than one body organ

☐ An abnormal lab result, physical exam finding or illness that is given many diagnoses or has no clear cause

ENVIRONMENT

☐ Someone in your neighborhood within 400 yards in any direction of your dwelling has been diagnosed with a tick borne infection [This includes vacation locations].

☐ You have someone living with you with any type of tick-borne infection—this assumes they were not merely tested for one infection. [It is not proven that the small Lyme-carrying ticks only carry Lyme, and it is possible some carry other infections without carrying Lyme at all.

☐ You have removed any ticks *from your body* in your lifetime at any location.

☐ You have removed ticks *from your clothing* in your lifetime at any location.

☐ After a tick or bug bite, you had a fever for at least 48 hours.

☐ After a tick or bug bite, you were ill.

☐ Grew up or played in areas with many small wild mammals

☐ When you are in a room that has visible mold or smells like mold and you start to feel ill, you do not return to your baseline health in 24 hours.

☐ Any discomfort *within two minutes* of being in a musty or moldy location. This may be a sign of chronic untreated infection, because a mere 30 inhalations of mold debris causes systemic effects in your body

☐ *Pets or farm animals* positive with ANY tick borne virus, bacteria or protozoa, or clinical symptoms without a clear diagnosis or cause

☐ The patient's **mother** is suspected of having or has been diagnosed with Babesia, Ehrlichia, Rocky Mountain Spotted Fever, Anaplasma, Lyme, Bartonella or other tick borne disease based on newer direct and indirect testing, or clinical signs and symptoms.

☐ **A sibling, father, spouse or child** with any tick borne infection

☐ **Casual or work-related exposure to outdoor environments** with brush, wild grasses, wild streams or woods (Examples- golf courses, parks, gardens, river banks, swamps, etc.)

☐ Pets, e.g., horses, dogs or cats, have had **outdoor exposures** to areas such as brush, wild grasses, wild streams or woods.

☐ You played in grass in the past.

☐ You have been bitten by fleas.

☐ You have been scratched by a cat or dog.

FINAL WORDS

Some of the above listed signs and symptoms fit other infections that may be more common than Lyme disease. Unfortunately, the research and experience indicating diverse infections carried by the Ixodes and other ticks is ignored so a small number of symptoms and signs were added to this checklist. . Further, "testing" usually involves one test for a mono-infection--Borrelia or Lyme. Ticks and other vectors should never be assumed to carry only Lyme disease.

Please note that when we are talking about the Ixodes tick we are *not* referring to this as a "deer tick" since it has over 200 vectors (Ostfeld). **Many of the tick reduction options presently suggested are not successful in accomplishing their goals.** Reducing deer populations, once thought to reduce tick populations and incidence of Lyme disease, may simply increase tick numbers in mammals and other carriers that live closer to humans.

All healers have their familiar way of thinking, testing and treating. Kuhn has shown we are all biased and struggle to be objective...and fail. Certainty is simply impossible in medical science. Further, tick and flea infections have almost infinite pathological effects because the human body and these clusters of infections are so complex. I have not suggested a grid or a set number of symptoms, because one would not fit this list. Simply, the goal of this checklist is to have you think broadly.

You cannot use this checklist to diagnose Lyme disease or to rule it out.

A Lyme checklist is very medically important, since it is still an emerging illness and can sometimes disable or increase mortality risk in patients of any age if not diagnosed and treated early in the infection.

Writings in the past fifteen years have either viewed Babesia and Bartonella as mere "co-infections," or a footnote of a spirochete infection [i.e., Lyme]. Either infection can hide for decades, and then possibly disable or kill a person by causing a clot, heart arrhythmia or by other means.

The detection of Lyme from stained tissue samples or blood is very difficult. Currently, the well-established indirect lab test patterns presented are not used or understood by all health care professionals. While this is fully understandable, I hope it may change in the coming decade. Tick infections have *systemic impacts* on the body, and are not limited to effects reported in journal articles, a few books or any national or international guidelines.

Dr. Schaller has published the four most recent textbooks on Babesia and the only recent textbook in any language on Bartonella. His most recent book on Lyme, Babesia and Bartonella includes a "researchers only" list of over 2,600 references considered to be **a start** for basic education in tick infection medicine.

He published articles on both Babesia as a cancer primer and Bartonella as a profound psychiatric disease under the supervision of the former editor of the *Journal of the American Medical Association (JAMA)*. He also published entries on multiple tick and flea-borne infections, including Babesia, Bartonella and Lyme disease, in a respected infection textbook endorsed by the NIH Director of Infectious Disease.

Dr. Schaller is the author of seven texts on tick and flea-borne infections. He is rated a BEST physician, an honor that is awarded to only 1 in 20 physicians by physician peers. He is also rated a TOP physician by patients, again ranking in the top 5 percent of physicians.

Copyright © 2011 JAMES SCHALLER, M.D., M.A.R. version 25.

This form may not be altered if it is printed or posted, in any manner, without written permission. It can be printed for free to assist in diagnostic reflections, as long as no line is redacted or altered, including the introduction or final paragraphs. Dr. Schaller does not claim that this is a flawless or final form, and defers all diagnostic decisions to your licensed health professional.

Bibliography (Lyme Disease)

Aalto A, Sjöwall J, Davidsson L, Forsberg P, Smedby O. Brain magnetic resonance imaging does not contribute to the diagnosis of chronic neuroborreliosis. Acta Radiol. 2007 Sep;48(7):755-62. PMID:17729007

Aberer E. [Neuroborreliosis or Borrelia hysteria. This case becomes a nightmare!].[Article in German]. MMW Fortschr Med. 2006 Nov 9;148(45):8. PMID:17615738

Aboul-Enein F, Kristoferitsch W. Normal pressure hydrocephalus or neuroborreliosis? Wien Med Wochenschr. 2009;159(1-2):58-61. PMID:19225737

Alaedini A, Latov N. Antibodies against OspA epitopes of Borrelia burgdorferi cross-react with neural tissue. J Neuroimmunol. 2005 Feb;159(1-2):192-5. Epub 2004 Nov 26. PMID:15652419

Angelakis E, Billeter SA, Breitschwerdt EB, Chomel BB, Raoult D. Potential for tick-borne bartonellosis. Emerg Infect Dis. 2010 Mar;16(3):385-91.

Auwaerter PG. Point: antibiotic therapy is not the answer for patients with persisting symptoms attributable to lyme disease. Clin Infect Dis. 2007 Jul 15;45(2):143-8. Epub 2007 Jun 5. PMID:17578771

Banarer M, Cost K, Rychwalski P, Bryant KA. Chronic lymphocytic meningitis in an adolescent. J Pediatr. 2005 Nov;147(5):686-90. PMID:16291364

Baneth G, Breitschwerdt EB, Hegarty BC, Pappalardo B, Ryan J. A survey of tick-borne bacteria and protozoa in naturally exposed dogs from Israel. Vet Parasitol. 1998 Jan 31;74(2-4):133-42.

Barbour AG. Laboratory aspects of Lyme borreliosis. Clin Microbiol Rev 1988 Oct;1(4):415-31.

Barie PS. Warning! Danger Will Robinson! Lyme disease clinical practice guidelines of the Infectious Diseases Society of America, activist patients, antitrust law, and prosecutorial zeal. Surg Infect (Larchmt). 2007 Apr;8(2):147-50. PMID:17437359

Batinac T, Petranovic D, Zamolo G, Petranovic D, Ruzic A. Lyme borreliosis and multiple sclerosis are associated with primary effusion lymphoma. Med Hypotheses. 2007;69(1):117-9. Epub 2007 Jan 2. PMID:17197115

Begon E. [Lyme arthritis, Lyme carditis and other presentations potentially associated to Lyme disease].[Article in French]. Med Mal Infect. 2007 Jul-Aug;37(7-8):422-34. Epub 2007 Aug 14. PMID:17698309

Benhnia MR, Wroblewski D, Akhtar MN, Patel RA, Lavezzi W, Gangloff SC, Goyert SM, Dvoráková J, Celer V. [Pharmacological aspects of Lyme borreliosis].[Article in Czech]. Ceska Slov Farm. 2004 Jul;53(4):159-64. PMID:15369225

Bhate C, Schwartz RA. Lyme disease: Part II. Management and prevention. J Am Acad Dermatol. 2011 Apr;64(4):639-53; quiz 654, 653. PMID:21414494

Biesiada G, Czapiel J, Sobczyk-Krupiarz I, Garlicki A, Mach T. Neuroborreliosis with extrapyramidal symptoms: a case report. Pol Arch Med Wewn. 2008 May;118(5):314-7. PMID:18619183

Billeter SA, Levy MG, Chomel BB, Breitschwerdt EB. Vector transmission of Bartonella species with emphasis on the potential for tick transmission. Med Vet Entomol. 2008 Mar;22(1):1-15.

Bitar I, Lally EV. Musculoskeletal manifestations of Lyme disease. Med Health R I. 2008 Jul;91(7):213-5. PMID:18705221

Blanc F. [Epidemiology of Lyme borreliosis and neuroborreliosis in France].[Article in French]. Rev Neurol (Paris). 2009 Aug-Sep;165(8-9):694-701. Epub 2009 May 17. PMID:19447458

Blanc F; GEBLY. [Neurologic and psychiatric manifestations of Lyme disease].[Article in French]. Med Mal Infect. 2007 Jul-Aug;37(7-8):435-45. Epub 2007 Mar 9. PMID:17350199

Bransfield RC, Wulfman JS, Harvey WT, Usman AI. The association between tick-borne infections, Lyme borreliosis and autism spectrum disorders. Med Hypotheses. 2008;70(5):967-74. Epub 2007 Nov 5. PMID:17980971

Brehm M, Rellecke P, Strauer BE. [Inflammatory cardiac diseases by primary extracardial diseases].[Article in German]. Internist (Berl). 2008 Jan;49(1):27-33. PMID:17992497

Breitschwerdt EB. Feline bartonellosis and cat scratch disease. Vet Immunol Immunopathol. 2008 May 15;123(1-2):167-71. Epub 2008 Jan 19. Review.

Breitschwerdt EB, Atkins CE, Brown TT, Kordick DL, Snyder PS. Bartonella vinsonii subsp. berkhoffii and related members of the alpha subdivision of the Proteobacteria in dogs with cardiac arrhythmias, endocarditis, or myocarditis. J Clin Microbiol. 1999 Nov;37(11):3618-26.

Breitschwerdt EB, Blann KR, Stebbins ME, Muñana KR, Davidson MG, Jackson HA, Willard MD. Clinicopathological abnormalities and treatment response in 24 dogs seroreactive to Bartonella vinsonii (berkhoffii) antigens. J Am Anim Hosp Assoc. 2004 Mar-Apr;40(2):92-101.

Breitschwerdt EB, Hegarty BC, Hancock SI. Sequential evaluation of dogs naturally infected with Ehrlichia canis, Ehrlichia chaffeensis, Ehrlichia equi, Ehrlichia ewingii, or Bartonella vinsonii. J Clin Microbiol. 1998 Sep;36(9):2645-51.

Breitschwerdt EB, Hegarty BC, Maggi R, Hawkins E, Dyer P. Bartonella species as a potential cause of epistaxis in dogs. J Clin Microbiol. 2005 May;43(5):2529-33.

Breitschwerdt EB, Kordick DL. Bartonellosis. J Am Vet Med Assoc. 1995 Jun 15;206(12):1928-31. Review.

Breitschwerdt EB, Kordick DL. Bartonella infection in animals: carriership, reservoir potential, pathogenicity, and zoonotic potential for human infection. Clin Microbiol Rev. 2000 Jul;13(3):428-38. Review.

Breitschwerdt EB, Kordick DL, Malarkey DE, Keene B, Hadfield TL, Wilson K. Endocarditis in a dog due to infection with a novel Bartonella subspecies. J Clin Microbiol. 1995 Jan;33(1):154-60.

Breitschwerdt EB, Maggi RG. A confusing case of canine vector-borne disease: clinical signs and progression in a dog co-infected with Ehrlichia canis and Bartonella vinsonii ssp. berkhoffii. Parasit Vectors. 2009 Mar 26;2 Suppl 1:S3.

Breitschwerdt EB, Maggi RG. Comparative medical features of canine and human bartonellosis. Clin Microbiol Infect. 2009 Dec;15 Suppl 2:106-7. Epub 2009 Apr 30.

Breitschwerdt EB, Maggi RG, Cadenas MB, de Paiva Diniz PP. A groundhog, a novel Bartonella sequence, and my father's death. Emerg Infect Dis. 2009 Dec;15(12):2080-6.

Breitschwerdt EB, Maggi RG, Chomel BB, Lappin MR. Bartonellosis: an emerging infectious disease of zoonotic importance to animals and human beings. J Vet Emerg Crit Care (San Antonio). 2010 Feb;20(1):8-30. Review.

Breitschwerdt EB, Maggi RG, Duncan AW, Nicholson WL, Hegarty BC, Woods CW. Bartonella species in blood of immunocompetent persons with animal and arthropod contact. Emerg Infect Dis. 2007 Jun;13(6):938-41.

Breitschwerdt EB, Maggi RG, Farmer P, Mascarelli PE. Molecular evidence of perinatal transmission of Bartonella vinsonii subsp. berkhoffii and Bartonella henselae to a child. J Clin Microbiol. 2010 Jun;48(6):2289-93. Epub 2010 Apr 14.

Breitschwerdt EB, Maggi RG, Lantos PM, Woods CW, Hegarty BC, Bradley JM. Bartonella vinsonii subsp. berkhoffii and Bartonella henselae bacteremia in a father and daughter with neurological disease. Parasit Vectors. 2010 Apr 8;3(1):29.

Breitschwerdt EB, Maggi RG, Nicholson WL, Cherry NA, Woods CW. Bartonella sp. bacteremia in patients with neurological and neurocognitive dysfunction. J Clin Microbiol. 2008 Sep;46(9):2856-61. Epub 2008 Jul 16.

Breitschwerdt EB, Maggi RG, Robert Mozayeni B, Hegarty BC, Bradley JM, Mascarelli PE. PCR amplification of Bartonella koehlerae from human blood and enrichment blood cultures. Parasit Vectors. 2010 Aug 24;3:76.

Breitschwerdt EB, Maggi RG, Sigmon B, Nicholson WL. Isolation of Bartonella quintana from a woman and a cat following putative bite transmission. J Clin Microbiol. 2007 Jan;45(1):270-2. Epub 2006 Nov 8.

Breitschwerdt EB, Maggi RG, Varanat M, Linder KE, Weinberg G. Isolation of Bartonella vinsonii subsp. berkhoffii genotype II from a boy with epithelioid hemangioendothelioma and a dog with hemangiopericytoma. J Clin Microbiol. 2009 Jun;47(6):1957-60. Epub 2009 Apr 15.

Breitschwerdt EB, Mascarelli PE, Schweickert LA, Maggi RG, Hegarty BC, Bradley JM, Woods CW. Hallucinations, sensory neuropathy, and peripheral visual deficits in a young woman infected with Bartonella koehlerae. J Clin Microbiol. 2011 Sep;49(9):3415-7. Epub 2011 Jul 6.

Breitschwerdt EB, Sontakke S, Cannedy A, Hancock SI, Bradley JM. Infection with Bartonella weissii and detection of Nanobacterium antigens in a North Carolina beef herd. J Clin Microbiol. 2001 Mar;39(3):879-82.

Breitschwerdt EB, Suksawat J, Chomel B, Hegarty BC. The immunologic response of dogs to Bartonella vinsonii subspecies berkhoffii antigens: as assessed by Western immunoblot analysis. J Vet Diagn Invest. 2003 Jul;15(4):349-54.

Brtkova J, Jirickova P, Kapla J, Dedic K,, Pliskova L. Borrelia arthritis and chronic myositis accompanied by typical chronic dermatitis. JBR-BTR. 2008 May-Jun;91(3):88-9. PMID:18661710

Burns RB, Hartman EE. A 58-year-old man with a diagnosis of chronic Lyme disease, 1 year later. JAMA. 2003 Dec 24;290(24):3247. PMID:14693878

Caimano MJ, Radolf JD, Sellati TJ. Signaling through CD14 attenuates the inflammatory response to Borrelia burgdorferi, the agent of Lyme disease. J Immunol. 2005 Feb 1;174(3):1539-48. PMID:15661914

Calza L, Manfredi R, Chiodo F. [Tick-borne infections].[Article in Italian]. Recenti Prog Med. 2004 Sep;95(9):403-13. PMID:15473378

Cameron D. Obstacles to trials of chronic Lyme disease in actual practice. Minerva Med. 2009 Oct;100(5):435-6. PMID:19910896

Cameron DJ. Clinical trials validate the severity of persistent Lyme disease symptoms. Med Hypotheses. 2009 Feb;72(2):153-6. Epub 2008 Nov 13. PMID:19013025

Cameron DJ. Proof that chronic lyme disease exists. Interdiscip Perspect Infect Dis. 2010;2010:876450. Epub 2010 May 25. PMID:20508824

Cerar T, Ruzic-Sabljic E, Cimperman J, Strle F. Comparison of immunofluorescence assay (IFA) and LIAISON in patients with different clinical manifestations of Lyme borreliosis. Wien Klin Wochenschr. 2006 Nov;118(21-22):686-90. PMID:17160608

Chandra A, Wormser GP, Klempner MS, Trevino RP, Crow MK, Latov N, Alaedini A. Anti-neural antibody reactivity in patients with a history of Lyme borreliosis and persistent symptoms. Brain Behav Immun. 2010 Aug;24(6):1018-24. Epub 2010 Mar 18th PMID:20227484

Chernogor LI, Arbatskaia EV, Danchinova GA, Kozlova IV, Gorina MO, Suntsova OV, Chaporgina EA, Belikov SI, Borisov VA. [Clinical and laboratory characterization of Ixodes tick-borne borreliosis in the Baikal area].[Article in Russian]. Zh Mikrobiol Epidemiol Immunobiol. 2005 Nov-Dec;(6):60-2. PMID:16438378

Chomel BB, Boulouis HJ, Maruyama S, Breitschwerdt EB. Bartonella spp. in pets and effect on human health. Emerg Infect Dis. 2006 Mar;12(3):389-94. PMID 16704774

Clarissou J, Song A, Bernedo C, Guillemot D, Dinh A, Ader F, Perronne C, Salomon J. Efficacy of a long-term antibiotic treatment in patients with a chronic Tick Associated Poly-organic Syndrome (TAPOS). Med Mal Infect. 2009 Feb;39(2):108-15. Epub 2009 Jan 4. PMID:19124209

Comer JA, Diaz T, Vlahov D, Monterroso E, Childs JE. Evidence of rodent-associated Bartonella and Rickettsia infections among intravenous drug users from Central and East Harlem, New York City. Am J Trop Med Hyg. 2001 Dec;65(6):855-60. PMID:11791987

Comer JA, Flynn C, Regnery RL, Vlahov D, Childs JE. Antibodies to Bartonella species in inner-city intravenous drug users in Baltimore, Md. Arch Intern Med. 1996 Nov 25;156(21):2491-5. PMID:8944742

Coyle PK. Lyme disease. In: Feldmann E, ed. Current diagnosis in neurology. St Louis:Mosby,1994; pp 110-4.

Coyle PK ed. Lyme Disease. St. Louis:Mosby Year Book 1993; pp 187-91.

Clark JR, Carlson RD, Sasaki CT, Pachner AR, Steere AC. Facial paralysis in Lyme disease. Laryngoscope 1985 Nov;95(11):1341-5.

Créange A. [Clinical manifestations and epidemiological aspects leading to a diagnosis of Lyme borreliosis: neurological and psychiatric manifestations in the course of Lyme borreliosis].[Article in French]. Med Mal Infect. 2007 Jul-Aug;37(7-8):532-9. Epub 2007 Mar 26. PMID:17368785

da Franca I, Santos L, Mesquita T, Collares-Pereira M, Baptista S, Vieira L, Viana I, Vale E, Prates C. Lyme borreliosis in Portugal caused by Borrelia lusitaniae? Clinical report on the first patient with a positive skin isolate. Wien Klin Wochenschr. 2005 Jun;117(11-12):429-32. PMID:16053200

Danz B, Kreft B, Radant K, Marsch WCh, Fiedler E. Skin-coloured facial oedema as an initial manifestation of acrodermatitis chronica atrophicans. J Eur Acad Dermatol Venereol. 2008 Jun;22(6):751-3. PMID:18482035

Dattwyler RJ, Halperin JJ, Volkman DJ, Luft BJ. Treatment of late Lyme borreliosis - randomized comparison of ceftriaxone and penicillin. Lancet 1988 May 28;1(8596):1191-4.

Dattwyler RJ, Luft BJ, Maladorno D, et al. Treatment of late Lyme disease - a comparison of 2 weeks vs 4 weeks of ceftriaxone. VII International Congress on Lyme Borreliosis. San Francisco, June, 1996.

Dattwyler RJ, Wormser GP, Rush TJ, Finkel MF, Schoen RT, Grunwaldt E, Franklin M, Hilton E, Bryant GL, Agger WA, Maladorno D. A comparison of two treatment regimens of ceftriaxone in late Lyme disease. Wien Klin Wochenschr. 2005 Jun;117(11-12):393-7. PMID:16053194 de Freitas MR. Infectious neuropathy. Curr Opin Neurol. 2007 Oct;20(5):548-52. PMID:17885443

De Heller-Milev M, Peter O, Panizzon RG, Laffitte E. [Borrelial erythema of the face].[Article in French]. Ann Dermatol Venereol. 2008 Dec;135(12):852-4. Epub 2008 Oct 26. PMID:19084697

DeLong A. Lyme disease. Med Health R I. 2008 Dec;91(12):390; author reply 390. PMID:19170319

DePietropaolo DL, Powers JH, Gill JM, Foy AJ. Diagnosis of Lyme disease. Del Med J. 2006 Jan;78(1):11-8. PMID:16548394

Dillon R, O'Connell S, Wright S. Lyme disease in the U.K.: clinical and laboratory features and response to treatment. Clin Med. 2010 Oct;10(5):454-7. PMID:21117376

Djukic M, Schmidt-Samoa C, Nau R, von Steinbüchel N, Eiffert H, Schmidt H. The diagnostic spectrum in patients with suspected chronic Lyme neuroborreliosis--the experience from one year of a university hospital's Lyme neuroborreliosis outpatients clinic. Eur J Neurol. 2011 Apr;18(4):547-55. Epub 2010 Oct 27. PMID:20977545

Drancourt M, Tran-Hung L, Courtin J, Lumley H, Raoult D. Bartonella quintana in a 4000-year-old human tooth. J Infect Dis. 2005 Feb 15;191(4):607-11.

Dressler F, Whalen JA, Reinhardt BN, Steere A. Western blotting in the serodiagnosis of Lyme disease. J Infect Dis 1993 Feb;167(2):392-400.

Egle UT. [Chronic borreliosis? No, psychosomatic illness! (interview by Dr. med. Brigitte Moreano)].[Article in German]. MMW Fortschr Med. 2005 May 26;147(21):15. PMID:15966166

Einecke U. [Winter pause was too short--ticks are already becoming mobile].[Article in German]. MMW Fortschr Med. 2008 Mar 13;150(11):12-4. PMID:18447267

Ekerfelt C, Andersson M, Olausson A, Bergström S, Hultman P. Mercury exposure as a model for deviation of cytokine responses in experimental Lyme arthritis: HgCl2 treatment decreases T helper cell type 1-like responses and arthritis severity but delays eradication of Borrelia burgdorferi in C3H/HeN mice. Clin Exp Immunol. 2007 Oct;150(1):189-97. Epub 2007 Aug 2. PMID:17672870

Emedicine Health. Lyme Disease Symptoms. http://www. emedicinehealth.com/lyme_disease/page3_em.htm#Lyme Disease Symptoms

Eskow E, Rao RV, Mordechai E. Concurrent infection of the central nervous system by Borrelia burgdorferi and Bartonella henselae: evidence for a novel tick-borne disease complex. Arch Neurol. 2001 Sep;58(9):1357-63.

Fallon BA, Levin ES, Schweitzer PJ, Hardesty D. Inflammation and central nervous system Lyme disease. Neurobiol Dis. March 2010, 37 (3) :534-41. Epub 2009 Nov 26. PMID:19944760

Fallon BA, Lipkin RB, Corbera KM, Yu S, Nobler MS, Keilp JG, Petkova E, Lisanby SH, Moeller JR, Slavov I, Van Heertum R, Mensh BD, Sackeim HA. Regional cerebral blood flow and metabolic rate in persistent Lyme encephalopathy. Arch Gen Psychiatry. 2009 May;66(5):554-63. PMID:19414715

Fallon BA, Nields JA. Lyme Disease: A Neuropsychiatric Illness. Am J Psychiatry 1994 Nov;151(11):1571-83. PMID:7943444

Feder HM Jr, Abeles M, Bernstein M, Whitaker-Worth D, Grant-Kels JM. Diagnosis, treatment, and prognosis of erythema migrans and Lyme arthritis. Clin Dermatol. 2006 Nov-Dec;24(6):509-20. PMID:17113969

Feder HM Jr , Gerber MA, Luger SW, Ryan SW. Persistence of serum antibodies to Borrelia burgdorferi in patients treated for Lyme disease. Clin Infect Dis 1992 Nov;15(5):788-93.

Feder HM Jr, Johnson BJ, O'Connell S, Shapiro ED, Steere AC, Wormser GP; Ad Hoc International Lyme Disease Group, Agger WA, Artsob H, Auwaerter P, Dumler JS, Bakken JS, Bockenstedt LK, Green J, Dattwyler RJ, Munoz J, Nadelman RB, Schwartz I, Draper T, McSweegan E, Halperin JJ, Klempner MS, Krause PJ, Mead P, Morshed M, Porwancher R, Radolf JD, Smith RP Jr, Sood S, Weinstein A, Wong SJ, Zemel L. A critical appraisal of "chronic Lyme disease". N Engl J Med. 2007 Oct 4;357(14):1422-30. PMID:17914043

Fingerle V, Huppertz HI. [Lyme borreliosis in children. Epidemiology, diagnosis, clinical treatment, and therapy].[Article in German]. Hautarzt. 2007 Jun;58(6):541-50, quiz 551-2. PMID:17729432

Fingerle V, Wilske B. [Stage-oriented treatment of Lyme borreliosis]. [Article in German]. MMW Fortschr Med. 2006 Jun 22;148(25):39-41. PMID:16859159

Finkel MJ, Halperin JJ. Nervous system Lyme neuroborreliosis revisited. Arch Neurol 1992 Jan;49(1):102-7.

Fomenko NV, Romanova EV, Mel'nikova OV, Chernousova NIa, Epikhina TI. [Detection of Borrelia DNA in the Borrelia burgdorferi sensu lato complex in the blood of patients with Ixodes tick-borne borrelios].[Article in Russian]. Klin Lab Diagn. 2006 Aug;(8):35-7. PMID:17087247

Fürst B, Glatz M, Kerl H, Müllegger RR. The impact of immunosuppression on erythema migrans. A retrospective study of clinical presentation, response to treatment and production of Borrelia antibodies in 33 patients. Clin Exp Dermatol. 2006 Jul;31(4):509-14. Erratum in Clin Exp Dermatol. 2006 Sep;31(5):751. PMID:16716151

Gheorghiev C, De Montleau F, Defuentes G. [Alcohol and epilepsy: a case report between alcohol withdrawal seizures and neuroborreliosis]. [Article in French]. Brain. 2011 Jun;37(3):231-7. Epub 2010 December 3. PMID:21703439

Ghosh S, Huber BT. Clonal diversification in OspA-specific antibodies from peripheral circulation of a chronic Lyme arthritis patient. J Immunol Methods. 2007 Apr 10;321(1-2):121-34. Epub 2007 Feb 6. PMID:17307198

Ghosh S, Seward R, Costello CE, Stollar BD, Huber BT. Autoantibodies from synovial lesions in chronic, antibiotic treatment-resistant Lyme arthritis bind cytokeratin-10. J Immunol. 2006 Aug 15;177(4):2486-94. PMID:16888010

Ghosh S, Steere AC, Stollar BD, Huber BT. In situ diversification of the antibody repertoire in chronic Lyme arthritis synovium. J Immunol. 2005 Mar 1;174(5):2860-9. PMID:15728496

Ginsberg L, Kidd D. Chronic and recurrent meningitis. Pract Neurol. 2008 Dec;8(6):348-61. PMID:19015295

Girschick HJ, Morbach H, Tappe D. Treatment of Lyme borreliosis. Arthritis Res Ther. 2009;11(6):258. Epub 2009 Dec 17. PMID:20067594

Gouveia EA, Alves MF, Mantovani E, Oyafuso LK, Bonoldi VL, Yoshinari NH. Profile of patients with Baggio-Yoshinari Syndrome admitted at "Instituto de Emilio Ribas Infectologia ". Rev Inst Med Trop Sao Paulo. 2010 Dec;52(6):297-303. PMID:21225212

Grabe HJ, Spitzer C, Luedemann J, Guertler L, Kramer A, John U, Freyberger HJ, Völzke H. No association of seropositivity for anti-Borrelia IgG antibody with mental and physical complaints. Nord J Psychiatry. 2008;62(5):386-91. PMID:18752103

Grygorczuk S, Hermanowska-Szpakowicz T, Kondrusik M, Pancewicz S, Zajkowska J. [Ehrlichiosis--a disease rarely recognized in Poland]. [Article in Polish]. Wiad Lek. 2004;57(9-10):456-61. PMID:15765762

Grygorczuk S, Pancewicz S, Zajkowska J, Kondrusik M, Moniuszko A. [Articular symptoms in Lyme borreliosis]. [Article in Polish]. Pol Merkur Lekarski. 2008 June: 24 (144) :542-4. PMID:18702339

Grygorczuk S, Pancewicz S, Zajkowska J, Kondrusik M, Swierzbińska R, Moniuszko A, Pawlak-Zalewska W. [Reinfection in Lyme borreliosis].[Article in Polish]. Pol Merkur Lekarski. 2008 Sep;25(147):257-9. PMID:19112844

Grygorczuk S, Zajkowska J, Panasiuk A, Kondrusik M, Chmielewski T, Swierzbińska R, Pancewicz S, Flisiak R, Tylewska-Wierzbanowska S. [Activity of the caspase-3 in the culture of peripheral blood mononuclear cells stimulated with Borrelia burgdorferi antigens]. [Article in Polish]. Przegl Epidemiol. 2008;62(1):85-91. PMID:18536229

Grygorczuk S, Zajkowska J, Swierzbińska R, Pancewicz S, Kondrusik M, Hermanowska-Szpakowicz T. [Concentrations of soluble factors participating in regulation of apoptosis of lymphocyte from patients with chronic lyme arthritis (preliminary report)].[Article in Polish]. Pol Merkur Lekarski. 2006 Jan;20(115):49-52. PMID:16617735

Hagberg L, Dotevall L. Neuroborreliosis with bad reputation. This is no mystical, difficult-to-treat infection!].[Article in Swedish]. Lakartidningen. 2007 Nov 28-Dec 4;104(48):3621-2. PMID:18193671

Halperin JJ. Prolonged Lyme disease treatment: enough is enough. Neurology. 2008 Mar 25;70(13):986-7. Epub 2007 Oct 10. PMID:17928578

Halperin JJ. Lyme Disease: An Evidence-Based Approach (Advances in Molecular and Cellular Biology Series). Wallingford, Oxfordshire, UK:CABI. 2011.

Halperin JJ, Krupp LB, Golightly MG, Volkman DJ. Lyme borreliosis-associated encephalopathy. Neurology 1990 Sep;40(9):1340-3.

Halperin JJ, Logigian EL, Finkel MF, Pearl RA. Practice parameters for the diagnosis of patients with nervous system Lyme borreliosis (Lyme disease). Neurology 1996 Mar;46(3):619-27. PMID:8618656

Halperin JJ, Shapiro ED, Logigian E, Belman AL, Dotevall L, Wormser GP, Krupp L, Gronseth G, Bever CT Jr; Quality Standards Subcommittee of the American Academy of Neurology. Practice parameter: treatment of nervous system Lyme disease (an evidence-based review): report of the Quality Standards Subcommittee of the American Academy of Neurology. Neurology. 2007 Jul 3;69(1):91-102. Epub 2007 May 23. Erratum in Neurology. 2008 Apr 1;70(14):1223. PMID:17522387

Hamblin T. Is chronic lymphocytic leukemia a response to infectious agents? Leuk Res. 2006 Sep;30(9):1063-4. Epub 2006 Jan 6. PMID:16406017

Hamlen R. Lyme borreliosis: perspective of a scientist-patient. Lancet Infect Dis. 2004 Oct;4(10):603-4. PMID:15451481

Hanses F, Audebert FX, Glück T, Salzberger B, Ehrenstein BP. [Suspected borreliosis - what's behind it?].[Article in German]. Dtsch Med Wochenschr. Aug 2011;136(33):1652-5. Epub 2011 Aug 10th PMID:21833884

Harrer T, Geissdörfer W, Schoerner C, Lang E, Helm G. Seronegative Lyme neuroborreliosis in a patient on treatment for chronic lymphatic leukemia. Infection. 2007 Apr;35(2):110-3. PMID:17401717

Hassler D, Schnauffer M, Ehrfeld H, Müller E. Disappearance of specific immune response after successful therapy of chronic Lyme borreliosis. Int J Med Microbiol. 2004 Apr;293 Suppl 37:161-4. PMID:15147000

Hausotter W. [Appraisal of Lyme borreliosis].[Article in German] Versicherungsmedizin. 2004 Mar 1;56(1):25-9. PMID:15049470

Hendrickx G, De Boeck H, Goossens A, Demanet C, Vandenplas Y. Persistent synovitis in children with Lyme arthritis: two unusual cases. An immunogenetic approach. Eur J Pediatr. 2004 Nov;163(11):646-50. Epub 2004 Jul 28. PMID:15503133

Hendrickx G, Demanet C, Vandenplas Y. Persistent synovitis in two children with Lyme arthritis linked with HLA-DRB1*1104. Eur J Pediatr. 2006 Jun;165(6):420-1. Epub 2006 Mar 4. PMID:16518608

Hodzic E, Feng S, Holden K, Freet KJ, Barthold SW. Persistence of Borrelia burgdorferi following antibiotic treatment in mice. Antimicrob Agents Chemother. 2008 May;52(5):1728-36. Epub 2008 Mar 3. PMID:18316520

Holmes KD. An appraisal of "chronic Lyme disease". N Engl J Med. 2008 Jan 24;358(4):429; author reply 430-1. PMID:18219749

Hoppa E, Bachur R. Lyme disease update. Curr Opin Pediatr. 2007 Jun;19(3):275-80. PMID:17505186

Horneff G. [Juvenile arthritides].[Article in German]. Z Rheumatol. 2010 Oct;69(8):719-35; quiz 736-7. PMID:20798949

Hospach T, Langendörfer M, Kalle TV, Tewald F, Wirth T, Dannecker GE. Mimicry of lyme arthritis by synovial hemangioma. Rheumatol Int. 2009 Dec 16. [Epub ahead of print] PMID:20013264

Hurley RA, Taber KH. Acute and chronic Lyme disease: controversies for neuropsychiatry. J Neuropsychiatry Clin Neurosci. 2008 Winter;20(1):iv-6. PMID:18305280

Hytönen J, Hartiala P, Oksi J, Viljanen MK. Borreliosis: recent research, diagnosis, and management. Scand J Rheumatol. 2008 May-Jun;37(3):161-72. PMID:18465449

The International Lyme and Associated Diseases Society (ILADS), Evidence-based guidelines for the management of Lyme disease. Expert Rev Anti-infect Ther, 2004. 2(Suppl): p. S1-S13.

Jacomo V, Kelly PJ, Raoult D (2002). Natural history of Bartonella infections (an exception to Koch's postulate). Clin Diagn Lab Immunol. 2002 Jan;9(1):8-18. PMID:11777823

Jakobs M, Morawietz L, Rothschenk H, Hopf T, Weiner S, Schausten
H, Krukemeyer

MG, Krenn V. [Synovitis score: value of histopathological diagnostics
in unclear arthritis.   Case reports from rheumatological pathological
practice].[Article in German]. Z Rheumatol. 2007 Dec;66(8):706-12.
PMID:18000669

Jarefors S, Janefjord CK, Forsberg P, Jenmalm MC, Ekerfelt C.
Decreased up-regulation of the interleukin-12Rbeta2-chain and
interferon-gamma secretion and increased number of forkhead box P3-
expressing cells in patients with a history of chronic Lyme borreliosis
compared with asymptomatic Borrelia-exposed individuals. Clin Exp
Immunol. 2007 Jan;147(1):18-27. PMID:17177959

Johnson BJ, Robbins KE, Bailey RE, Cao BL, Sviat SL, Craven RB,
Mayer LW, Dennis DT. Serodiagnosis of Lyme disease: Accuracy of a
two-step approach using a flagella-based ELISA and immunoblotting.
J Infect Dis 1996 Aug;174(2):346-53. PMID:8699065

Johnson L, Aylward A, Stricker RB. Healthcare access and burden
of care for patients with Lyme disease: a large United States
survey. Health Policy. 2011 Sep;102(1):64-71. Epub 2011 Jun 14.
PMID:21676482

Johnson M, Feder HM Jr. Chronic Lyme disease: a survey of
Connecticut primary care physicians. J Pediatr. 2010 Dec;157(6):1025-
1029. e1-2. Epub 2010 Sep 1. PMID:20813379

Kaiser R. [Clinical courses of acute and chronic neuroborreliosis
following treatment with ceftriaxone].[Article in German]. Nervenarzt.
2004 Jun;75(6):553-7. PMID:15257378

Kalac M, Suvic-Krizanic V, Ostojic S, Kardum-Skelin I, Barsic
B, Jaksica B. Central nervous system involvement of previously
undiagnosed chronic lymphocytic leukemia in a patient with
neuroborreliosis. Int J Hematol. 2007 May;85(4):323-5.
PMID:17483076

Kaminsky A. Erythema figuratum. [Article in English, Spanish].
Proceedings Dermosifiliogr. 2009 Dec;100 Suppl 2:88-109.
PMID:20096167

Kaplan FR, Jones-Woodward L. Lyme encephalopathy: a
neuropsychological perspective. Semin Neurol 1997 Mar;17(1):31-7.

Karlsson M, Hovind-Hougen K, Svenungsson B, Stiernstedt G.
Cultivation and characterization of spirochetes from cerebrospinal
fluid of patients with Lyme borreliosis. J Clin Microbiol 1990
Mar;28(3):473-9.

Katchanov J, Siebert E, Klingebiel R, Endres M. Infectious
vasculopathy of intracranial large- and medium-sized vessels in
neurological intensive care unit: a clinical-radiological study. Neurocrit
Care. 2010 Jun;12(3):369-74. PMID:20146025

Keller TL, Halperin JJ, Whitman M. PCR detection of Borrelia
burgdorferi DNA in cerebrospinal fluid of Lyme neuroborreliosis
patients. Neurology 1992 Jan;42(1):32-42.

Kemperman MM, Bakken JS, Kravitz GR. Dispelling the
chronic Lyme disease myth. Minn Med. 2008 Jul;91(7):37-41.
PMID:18714930

Kestelyn PG. An eye on inflammatory eye disease. Acta Clin Belg.
2005 Sep-Oct;60(5):270-5. PMID:16398326

Kisand KE, Prükk T, Kisand KV, Lüüs SM, Kalbe I, Uibo R.
Propensity to excessive proinflammatory response in chronic Lyme
borreliosis. APMIS. 2007 Feb;115(2):134-41. PMID:17295680

Kiser, K. In the Lyme light. Minn Med. 2009 Nov;92(11):10-2.
PMID:20069988

Klimkiewicz Wolańska-E, Szymanska J, Bachanek T. Orofacial
symptoms related to boreliosis--case report. Agric Environ Med Ann.
2010 Dec;17(2):319-21. PMID:21186776

Kohler J, Kern U, Kasper J, Rhese-Kupper B, Thoden U. Chronic central nervous system involvement in Lyme borreliosis. Neurology 1988 Jun;38(6):863-7.

Kordick DL, Breitschwerdt EB. Intraerythrocytic presence of Bartonella henselae. J Clin Microbiol. 1995 Jun;33(6):1655-6.

Kordick DL, Breitschwerdt EB. Relapsing bacteremia after blood transmission of Bartonella henselae to cats. Am J Vet Res. 1997 May;58(5):492-7.

Kordick DL, Breitschwerdt EB. Persistent infection of pets within a household with three Bartonella species. Emerg Infect Dis. 1998 Apr-Jun;4(2):325-8.

Kordick SK, Breitschwerdt EB, Hegarty BC, Southwick KL, Colitz CM, Hancock SI, Bradley JM, Rumbough R, Mcpherson JT, MacCormack JN. Coinfection with multiple tick-borne pathogens in a Walker Hound kennel in North Carolina. J Clin Microbiol. 1999 Aug;37(8):2631-8.

Krause A, Fingerle V. [Lyme borreliosis].[Article in German]. Z Rheumatol. 2009 May;68(3):239-52, quiz 253-4. PMID:19387665

Krause A, Herzer P. [Early diagnosis of Lyme arthritis].[Article in German]. Z Rheumatol. 2005 Nov;64(8):531-7. PMID:16328757

Kremer S, Holl N, Schmitt E, De Sèze J, Moser T, Dieterich JL Mann. [Imaging of non-traumatic and non-tumoral cord lesions]. [Article in French]. J Radiol. 2010 Sep;91(9 Pt 2):969-87. PMID:20814389

Kruger H, Kohlhepp W, Konig S. Follow-up of antibiotically treated and untreated neuroborreliosis. Acta Neurol Scand 1990 Jul;82(1):59-67.

Krupp LB. Lyme disease. In: Samuels MA, Feske S, eds. Office practice of neurology. London:Churchill-Livingstone, 1996; pp 383-7.

Kuenzle S, von Büdingen HC, Meier M, Harrer MD, Urich E, Becher B, Goebels N. Pathogen specificity and autoimmunity are distinct features of antigen-driven immune responses in neuroborreliosis. Infect Immun. 2007 Aug;75(8):3842-7. Epub 2007 May 21. PMID:17517881

Kuhn TS. The structures of scientific revolutions. Chicago: University Of Chicago Press; 3rd edition;1996. Summarized: http://des.emory. edu/mfp/Kuhn.html

LaFleur RL, Dant JC, Wasmoen TL, Callister SM, Jobe DA, Lovrich SD, Warner TF, Abdelmagid OR, Schell RF. Bacterin that induces anti-OspA and anti-OspC borreliacidal antibodies provides a high level of protection against canine Lyme disease. Clin Vaccine Immunol. 2009 Feb;16(2):253-9. Epub 2008 Dec 3. PMID:19052162

Lantos PM. Chronic Lyme disease: the controversies and the science. Expert Rev Anti Infect Ther. 2011 Jul;9(7):787-97. PMID:21810051

Lappin MR, Breitschwerdt E, Brewer M, Hawley J, Hegarty B, Radecki S. Prevalence of Bartonella species antibodies and Bartonella species DNA in the blood of cats with and without fever. J Feline Med Surg. 2009 Feb;11(2):141-8. Epub 2008 Aug 29.

Lee G, Xiang Z, Brannagan TH 3rd, Chin RL, Latov N. Differential gene expression in chronic inflammatory demyelinating polyneuropathy (CIDP) skin biopsies. J Neurol Sci. 2010 Mar 15;290(1-2):115-22. Epub 2009 Nov 17. PMID:19922956

Lesnicar G, Zerdoner D. Temporomandibular joint involvement caused by Borrelia Burgdorferi. J Craniomaxillofac Surg. 2007 Dec;35(8):397-400. Epub 2007 Oct 17. PMID:17942315

Leverkus M., Finner AM, Pokrywka A, Franke I, Gollnick H. Metastatic squamous cell carcinoma of the ankle in long-standing untreated acrodermatitis chronica atrophicans. Dermatology. 2008;217(3):215-8. Epub 2008 Jul 8. PMID:18607109

Liang FT, Brown EL, Wang T, Iozzo RV, Fikrig E. Protective niche for Borrelia burgdorferi to evade humoral immunity. Am J Pathol. 2004 Sep;165(3):977-85. PMID:15331421

Lins H, Wallesch CW, Wunderlich MT. Sequential analyses of neurobiochemical markers of cerebral damage in cerebrospinal fluid and serum in CNS infections. Acta Neurol Scand. 2005 Nov;112(5):303-8. PMID:16218912

Listernick R. A 17-year-old boy previously diagnosed with chronic Lyme disease. Patient complained of low-grade fevers, headaches, pharyngitis, and suspected his mother was trying to poison him. Pediatr Ann. 2004 Aug;33(8):494-8. PMID:15354601

Ljøstad U, Mygland A. [Lyme borreliosis in adults].[Article in Norwegian]. Tidsskr Nor Laegeforen. 2008 May 15;128(10):1175-8. PMID:18480867

Ljøstad U, Mygland A. Remaining complaints 1 year after treatment for acute Lyme neuroborreliosis; frequency, pattern and risk factors. Eur J Neurol. 2010 Jan;17(1):118-23. Epub 2009 Jul 23. PMID:19645771

Logigian EL. Neurologic manifestations of Lyme disease. In: Rahn QW, Evans J, eds. Lyme disease. Philadelphia:ACP, 1998; pp 89-106.

Logigian EL, Kaplan RF, Steere AC. Chronic neurologic manifestations of Lyme disease. N Engl J Med 1990 Nov;323(21):1438-44.

Lu B, PereiraPerrin M. A novel immunoprecipitation strategy identifies a unique functional mimic of the glial cell line-derived neurotrophic factor family ligands in the pathogen Trypanosoma cruzi. Infect Immun. 2008 Aug, 76 (8) :3530-8. Epub 2008 Jun 9. PMID:18541656

Lukashova LV, Karpova MR, Pirogova NP, Kiiutsina TA, Lepekhin AV, Perevozchikova TV, Faĭt EA. [Functional status of peripheral blood monocyte in patients with Ixodes tick-borne borreliosis accompanied by opisthorchiasis].[Article in Russian]. Zh Mikrobiol Epidemiol Immunobiol. 2006 Mar-Apr;(2):81-3. PMID:16758907

Maco V, Maguiña C, Tirado A, Maco V, Vidal JE. Carrion's disease (Bartonellosis bacilliformis) confirmed by histopathology in the High Forest of Peru. Rev Inst Med Trop Sao Paulo. 2004 May-Jun;46(3):171-4. PMID:15286824

Maggi RG, Breitschwerdt EB. Isolation of bacteriophages from Bartonella vinsonii subsp. berkhoffii and the characterization of Pap31 gene sequences from bacterial and phage DNA. J Mol Microbiol Biotechnol. 2005;9(1):44-51.

Maggi RG, Breitschwerdt EB. Potential limitations of the 16S-23S rRNA intergenic region for molecular detection of Bartonella species. J Clin Microbiol. 2005 Mar;43(3):1171-6.

Maloney E. Chronic lyme disease counterpoint. Minn Med. 2008 Aug;91(8):6-7. PMID:18773702

Maloney EL. An appraisal of "chronic Lyme disease". N Engl J Med. 2008 Jan 24;358(4):428-9; author reply 430-1. PMID:18219748

Maloney EL. Article shed no light. Minn Med. 2010 Jan;93(1):6-7. PMID:20191722

Markeljević J, Sarac H, Rados M. Tremor, seizures and psychosis as presenting symptoms in a patient with chronic Lyme neuroborreliosis (LNB). Coll Antropol. 2011 Jan;35 Suppl 1:313-8. PMID:21648354

Marques A. Chronic Lyme disease: a review. Infect Dis Clin North Am. 2008 Jun;22(2):341-60, vii-viii. PMID:18452806

Martí-Martínez S, Martín-Estefanía C, Turpín-Fenoll L, Pampliega-Pérez A, Reus-Bañuls S, García-Barragán N, Villarubia-Lor B. [Bilateral papilloedema as the initial symptom of POEMS syndrome]. [Article in Spanish]. Rev Neurol. 2006 Nov 1-15;43(9):531-4. PMID:17072808

Mayer L, Merz S. An appraisal of "chronic Lyme disease". Engl J Med. 2008 Jan 24;358(4):428; author reply 430-1. PMID:18216368

Mayo Clinic Staff. Lyme Disease Symptoms. http://www.mayoclinic.com/health/lyme-disease/DS00116/DSECTION=symptoms

McGill S, Hjelm E, Rajs J, Lindquist O, Friman G. Bartonella spp. antibodies in forensic samples from Swedish heroin addicts. Ann N Y Acad Sci. 2003 Jun;990:409-13. PMID:12860665

Mervin P. Don't deny treatment. Minn Med. 2009 Dec;92(12):6. PMID:20092159

Michau TM, Breitschwerdt EB, Gilger BC, Davidson MG. Bartonella vinsonii subspecies berkhoffi as a possible cause of anterior uveitis and choroiditis in a dog. Vet Ophthalmol. 2003 Dec;6(4):299-304.

Michel JM, Sellal F. ["Reversible" dementia in 2011].[Article in French]. Old Geriatr Psychol neuropsychiatrist. 2011 Jun;9(2):211-25. PMID:21690030

Miklossy J. Chronic inflammation and amyloidogenesis in Alzheimer's disease -- role of Spirochetes. J Alzheimers Dis. 2008 May;13(4):381-91. PMID:18487847

Miklossy J, Kasas S, Zurn AD, McCall S, Yu S, McGeer PL. Persisting atypical and cystic forms of Borrelia burgdorferi and local inflammation in Lyme neuroborreliosis. J Neuroinflammation. 2008 Sep 25;5:40. PMID:18817547

Miklossy J, Khalili K, Gern L, Ericson RL, Darekar P, Bolle L, Hurlimann J, Paster BJ. Borrelia burgdorferi persists in the brain in chronic lyme neuroborreliosis and may be associated with Alzheimer disease. J Alzheimers Dis. 2004 Dec;6(6):639-49; discussion 673-81. PMID:15665404

Miller JC, von Lackum K, Woodman ME, Stevenson B. Detection of Borrelia burgdorferi gene expression during mammalian infection using transcriptional fusions that produce green fluorescent protein. Microb Pathog. 2006 Jul;41(1):43-7. Epub 2006 May 24. PMID:16723206

Mitty J, Margolius D. Updates and controversies in the treatment of Lyme disease. Med Health R I. 2008 Jul;91(7):219, 222-3. PMID:18705223

Moniuszko A, Czupryna P, Zajkowska J, Pancewicz SA, Grygorczuk S, Kondrusik M. [Post Lyme syndrome as a clinical problem]. [Article in Polish]. Pol Merkur Lekarski. 2009 Mar;26(153):227-30. PMID:19388538

Morales SC, Breitschwerdt EB, Washabau RJ, Matise I, Maggi RG, Duncan AW. Detection of Bartonella henselae DNA in two dogs with pyogranulomatous lymphadenitis. J Am Vet Med Assoc. 2007 Mar 1;230(5):681-5.

Mosbacher M, Elliott SP, Shehab Z, Pinnas JL, Klotz JH, Klotz SA. Cat scratch disease and arthropod vectors: more to it than a scratch? J Am Board Fam Med. 2010 Sep-Oct;23(5):685-6. PMID:20823366

Mulleger RR, Millner MM, Stanek, Spork KD. Penicillin G and ceftriaxone in the treatment of neuroborreliosis in children - a prospective study. Infection 1991 Jul-Aug;19(4):279-83.

Mygland A, Skarpaas T, Ljøstad U. Chronic polyneuropathy and Lyme disease. Eur J Neurol. 2006 Nov;13(11):1213-5. PMID:17038034

Nadelman RB, Arlen Z, Wormser GP. Life threatening complications of empiric ceftriaxone for 'seronegative' Lyme disease. South Med J 1991 Oct;84(10):1263-5.

Nafeev AA Klimova LV. [Clinical manifestations of neuroborreliosis in the Volga region].[Article in Russian]. Ter Arkh. 2010;82(11):68-70. PMID:21381354

Narayan K, Dail D, Li L, Cadavid D, Amrute S, Fitzgerald-Bocarsly P, Pachner AR. The nervous system as ectopic germinal center: CXCL13 and IgG in lyme neuroborreliosis. Ann Neurol. 2005 Jun;57(6):813-23. PMID:15929033

Nau R, Christian HJ, Eiffert H. Lyme disease--current state of knowledge. Dtsch Arztebl Int. 2009 Jan;106(5):72-81, 82 quiz, I. Epub 2009 Jan 30. PMID:19562015

Nigrovic LE, Thompson KM. The Lyme vaccine: a cautionary tale. Epidemiol Infect. 2007 Jan;135(1):1-8. Epub 2006 Aug 8. PMID:16893489

[No authors listed] [Differential aspects of multiple sclerosis and chronic borrelial encephalomyelitis].[Article in Russian]. Nevrol Zh Im SS Korsakova Psikhiatr. 2011;111(7):8-12. PMID:21947065

Nocton JJ, Bloom BJ, Rutledge BJ, Logigian EL, Schmid CH, Steere AC. Detection of Borrelia burgdorferi DNA by polymerase chain reaction in cerebrospinal fluid in Lyme neuroborreliosis. J Infect Dis 1996 Sep;174(3):623-7.

Nygård K, Brantsaeter AB, Mehl R. Disseminated and chronic Lyme borreliosis in Norway, 1995 - 2004. Euro Surveill. 2005 Oct;10(10):235-8. PMID:16282646

Ogrinc K, Logar M, Lotric-Furlan S, Cerar D, Ruzić-Sabljić E, Strle F. Doxycycline versus ceftriaxone for the treatment of patients with chronic Lyme borreliosis. Wien Klin Wochenschr. 2006 Nov;118(21-22):696-701. PMID:17160610

Oksi J, Nikoskelainen J, Hiekkanen H, Lauhio A, Peltomaa M, Pitkäranta A, Nyman D, Granlund H, Carlsson SA, Seppälä I, Valtonen V, Viljanen M. Duration of antibiotic treatment in disseminated Lyme borreliosis: a double-blind, randomized, placebo-controlled, multicenter clinical study. Eur J Clin Microbiol Infect Dis. 2007 Aug;26(8):571-81. PMID:17587070

Ostendorf GM. [No work disability in supposed post-borreliosis syndrome. On the decision of the OLG Saarbrücken of 19 May 2010]. [Article in German].Versicherungsmedizin. 2011 Jun 1;63(2):106-7. PMID:21698949

Ostfeld RS. Lyme Disease: The Ecology of a Complex System. New York: Oxford University Press. 2011

Pachner AR. Lyme neuroborreliosis. In: Johnson RT, Griffin JW, eds. Current therapy in neurologic disease. St Louis: Mosby, 1997; pp 140-6.

Pachner AR, Delaney E. The polymerase chain reaction in the diagnosis of Lyme neuroborreliosis. Ann Neurol 1993 Oct;34(4):544-50.

Pachner AR, Duray P, Steere AC. Central nervous system manifestations of Lyme disease. Arch Neurol. 1989 Jul;46(7):790-5.

Pachner AR, Steere AC. The triad of neurologic manifestations of Lyme disease: meningitis, cranial neuritis, and radiculoneuritis. Neurology. 1985 Jan;35(1):47-53.

Pancewicz S, Popko J, Rutkowski R, Knaś M, Grygorczuk S, Guszczyn T, Bruczko M, Szajda S, Zajkowska J, Kondrusik M, Sierakowski S, Zwierz K. Activity of lysosomal exoglycosidases in serum and synovial fluid in patients with chronic Lyme and rheumatoid arthritis. Scand J Infect Dis. 2009;41(8):584-9. PMID:19513935

Papo T. [Could aspecific symptoms be related to Borrelia infection?].
[Article in French]. Med Mal Infect. 2007 Jul-Aug;37(7-8):507-10.
Epub 2007 Mar 13. PMID:17360137

Parish JM. Sleep-related problems in common medical conditions.
Chest. 2009 Feb;135(2):563-72. PMID:19201722

Parker M, Turhan V, Aslan M, Musellim B, Hot Topic Y, Ertugrul
B. [First report of three culture confirmed human Lyme cases in
Turkey].[Article in Turkish]. Find Antimicrob. 2010 Jan;44(1):133-9.
PMID:20455410

Persecǎ T, Feder A, Molnar GB. [Results of etiologic diagnosis in
clinical syndrome consistent with acute and chronic borreliosis].
[Article in Romanian]. Rev Med Chir Soc Med Nat Iasi. 2008 Apr-
Jun;112(2):496-501. PMID:19295026

Pfister HW. [Clinical aspects of neuroborreliosis].[Article in
German]. MMW Fortschr Med. 2010 Jul 1;152(25-27):31-4; quiz 35.
PMID:20672660

Pfister HW, Rupprecht TA. Clinical aspects of neuroborreliosis and
post-Lyme disease syndrome in adult patients. Int J Med Microbiol.
2006 May;296 Suppl 40:11-6. Epub 2006 Mar 9. PMID:16524775

Phillips SE, Burrascano JJ, Harris NS, Johnson L, Smith PV, Stricker
RB. Chronic infection in 'post-Lyme borreliosis syndrome'. Int J
Epidemiol. 2005 Dec;34(6):1439-40; author reply 1440-3. Epub 2005
Nov 30. PMID:16319107

Pourel J. [Clinical diagnosis of Lyme borreliosis in case of joint and
muscular presentations].[Article in French]. Med Mal Infect. 2007 Jul-
Aug;37(7-8):523-31. Epub 2007 Mar 26. PMID:17368783

Przytuła L, Gińdzieńska-Sieśkiewicz E, Sierakowski S. [Diagnosis
and treatment of Lyme arthritis].[Article in Polish]. Przegl Epidemiol.
2006;60 Suppl 1:125-30. PMID:16909789

Puéchal X. [Non antibiotic treatments of Lyme borreliosis].[Article in French]. Med Mal Infect. 2007 Jul-Aug;37(7-8):473-8. Epub 2007 Mar 21. PMID:17376627

Puius YA, Kalish RA. Lyme arthritis: pathogenesis, clinical presentation, and management. Infect Dis Clin North Am. 2008 Jun;22(2):289-300, vi-vii. PMID:18452802

Reik L Jr. Lyme Disease and the Nervous System. New York:Thieme Medical Publishers. 1991, pp 57-61.

Reik L Jr. Neurologic aspects of North American Lyme disease. In Lyme Disease, ed. Patricia K. Coyle, M.D. St. Louis:Mosby-Year Book Inc. 1993, pp.101-112.

Renaud I, Cachin C, Gerster JC. Good outcomes of Lyme arthritis in 24 patients in an endemic area of Switzerland. Joint Bone Spine. 2004 Jan;71(1):39-43. PMID:14769519

Reshetova GG, Zaripova TN, Titskaia EV, Moskvin VS, Udintsev SN. [Physical factors in rehabilitation treatment of patients with Ixodes tick-borne borreliosis with primary lesions of the joints]. [Article in Russian]. Vopr Kurortol Fizioter Lech Fiz Kult. 2004 Nov-Dec;(6):10-3. PMID:15717529

Roche Lanquetot MO, Ader F, Durand MC, Carlier R, Defferriere H, Dinh A, Herrmann JL, Guillemot D, Perrone C, Salomon J. [Results of a prospective standardized study of 30 patients with chronic neurological and cognitive disorders after tick bites].[Article in French]. Med Mal Infect. 2008 Oct;38(10):543-8. PMID:18722064

Rolain JM, Brouqui P, Koehler JE, Maguina C, Dolan MJ, Raoult D. Recommendations for treatment of human infections caused by Bartonella species. Antimicrob Agents Chemother. 2004 Jun;48(6):1921-33. PMID:15155180

Rorat M, Kuchar E, Szenborn L, Małyszczak K. [Growing boreliosis anxiety and its reasons].[Article in Polish]. Psychiatr Pol 2010 Nov-Dec;44(6):895-904. PMID:21449171

Rossi M. [Late manifestations of Lyme borreliosis].[Article in German]. Ther Umsch. 2005 Nov;62(11):745-9. PMID:16350537

Roth J, Scheer I, Kraft S, Keitzer R, Riebel T. Uncommon synovial cysts in children. Eur J Pediatr. 2006 Mar;165(3):178-81. Epub 2005 Dec 13. PMID:16344992

Rudenko N, Golovchenko M, Růzek D, Piskunova N, Mallátová N, Grubhoffer L. Molecular detection of Borrelia bissettii DNA in serum samples from patients in the Czech Republic with suspected borreliosis. FEMS Microbiol Lett. March 2009, 292 (2) :274-81. Epub 2009 Jan 28. PMID:19187198

Samuels DS, Radolf JD, eds. Borrelia: Molecular Biology, Host Interaction and Pathogenesis. Norfolk, UK: Caister Academic Press. 2010.

Savely VR. Update on lyme disease: the hidden epidemic. Brews J Nurs. 2008 Jul-Aug;31(4):236-40. PMID:18641487

Savely V. Lyme disease: a diagnostic dilemma. Nurse Pract. 2010 Jul;35(7):44-50. PMID:20555245

Schaller J. The Diagnosis, Treatment and Prevention of Bartonella: Atypical Bartonella Treatment Failures and 40 Hypothetical Physical Exam Findings – Full Color Edition. Volume I-II. Tampa, FL:Hope Academic Press. 2008.

Schaller J. Babesia. in Encyclopedia of Plagues, Pestilence and Pandemics. Ed. J. Bryre. Westport, CT: Greenwood Press; 2008.

Schaller J. Bartonella. in Encyclopedia of Plagues, Pestilence and Pandemics. Ed. J. Bryre, Westport, CT: Greenwood Press; 2008

Schaller J. Lyme Disease. in Encyclopedia of Plagues, Pestilence and Pandemics. Ed. J. Bryre. Westport, CT: Greenwood Press; 2008

Schaller J. Babesia 2009 Supplement and Update. Tampa, FL:Hope Academic Press. 2009.

Schaller JL. Artemisin, Artesunate, Artemisinic Acid and Other Derivatives of Artemisia Used for Malaria, Babesia and Cancer. Tampa, FL: Hope Academic Press. 2006.

Schaller JL. The Health Care Professional's Guide to the Treatment and Diagnosis of Human Babesiosis, An Extensive Review of New Human Species and Advanced Treatments. Tampa, FL: Hope Academic Press. 2006.

Schaller JL, Burkland GA. Case report: rapid and complete control of idiopathic hypereosinophilia with imatinib mesylate. MedGenMed. 2001;3(5):9.

Schaller JL, Burkland GA, Langhoff PJ. Are various Babesia species a missed cause for hypereosinophilia? A follow-up on the first reported case of imatinib mesylate for idiopathic hypereosinophilia. MedGenMed. 2007 Feb 27;9(1):38.

Schaller JL, Burkland GA, Langhoff PJ. Do bartonella infections cause agitation, panic disorder, and treatment-resistant depression? MedGenMed. 2007 Sep 13;9(3):54.

Scheffer RE, Linden S. Concurrent medical conditions with pediatric bipolar disorder. Curr Opin Psychiatry. 2007 Jul;20(4):398-401. PMID:17551356

Schnarr S, Franz JK, Krause A, Zeidler H. Infection and musculoskeletal conditions: Lyme borreliosis. Best Pract Res Clin Rheumatol. 2006 Dec;20(6):1099-118. PMID:17127199

Schutzer SE, Angel TE, Liu T, Schepmoes AA, TR Clauss, JN Adkins, DG Camp, Holland BK, Bergquist J, Coyle PK, Smith RD, Fallon BA, Natelson BH. Distinct cerebrospinal fluid proteomes differentiate post-treatment lyme disease from chronic fatigue syndrome. PLoS One. 2011 Feb 23;6(2):e17287. PMID:21383843

Schweighofer CD, Fätkenheuer G, Staib P, Hallek M, Reiser M. Lyme disease in a patient with chronic lymphocytic leukemia mimics leukemic meningeosis. Onkologie. 2007 Nov;30(11):564-6. Epub 2007 Oct 16. PMID:17992027

Science Daily (Jan 6, 2009). New Bartonella Species That Infects Humans Discovered. Available at http://www.sciencedaily.com/releases/2009/01/090106145006.htm

Shapiro ED. Tick-borne diseases. Adv Pediatr Infect Dis. 1997;13:187-218. Review.

Shapiro ED. Long-term outcomes of persons with Lyme disease. Vector Borne Zoonotic Dis. 2002 Winter;2(4):279-81.

Shapiro ED, Gerber MA. Lyme disease and facial nerve palsy. Arch Pediatr Adolesc Med. 1997 Dec;151(12):1183-4.

Sherr VT. Human babesiosis--an unrecorded reality. Absence of formal registry undermines its detection, diagnosis and treatment, suggesting need for immediate mandatory reporting. Med Hypotheses. 2004;63(4):609-15. PMID:15325004

Sherr VT. Munchausen's syndrome by proxy and Lyme disease: medical misogyny or diagnostic mystery? Med Hypotheses. 2005;65(3):440-7. PMID:15925450

Siegel DM. Chronic arthritis in adolescence. Adolesc Med State Art Rev. 2007 May;18(1):47-61, viii. PMID:18605390

Sigal LH. Summary of the first 100 patients seen at a Lyme disease referral center. Am J Med 1990 Jun;88(6):577-83. PMID:2346158

Sigal LH. Current recommendations for the treatment of Lyme disease. Drugs 1992 May;43(5):683-99. PMID:1379147

Sigal LH. Long-term consequences of Lyme disease. In: Rahn QW, Evans J, eds. Lyme disease. Philadelphia:ACP, 1998; pp 137-53.

Sigal LH, Hassett AL. Commentary: 'What's in a name? That which we call a rose by any other name would smell as sweet.' Shakespeare W. Romeo and Juliet, II, ii(47-48). Int J Epidemiol. 2005 Dec;34(6):1345-7. Epub 2005 Sep 2. PMID:16143662

Simakova AI, Popov AF, Dadalova OB. [Ixodes tick-borne borreliosis with erythema nodosum].[Article in Russian]. Med Parazitol (Mosk). 2005 Oct-Dec;(4):31-2. PMID:16445235

Sjöwall J, Carlsson A, Vaarala O, Bergström S, Ernerudh J, Forsberg P, Ekerfelt C. Innate immune responses in Lyme borreliosis: enhanced tumour necrosis factor-alpha and interleukin-12 in asymptomatic individuals in response to live spirochetes. Clin Exp Immunol. 2005 Jul;141(1):89-98. PMID:15958074

Skotarczak B. Canine ehrlichiosis. Ann Agric Environ Med. 2003;10(2):137-41. PMID:14677903

Smith HM, Reporter R, Rood MP, Linscott AJ, Mascola LM, Hogrefe W, Purcell RH. Prevalence study of antibody to ratborne pathogens and other agents among patients using a free clinic in downtown Los Angeles. J Infect Dis. 2002 Dec 1;186(11):1673-6. PMID:12447746

Smith IS, Rechlin DP. Delayed diagnosis of neuroborreliosis presenting as bell palsy and meningitis. J Am Osteopath Assoc. 2010 Aug;110(8):441-4. PMID: 20805550

Sobek V, Birkner N, Falk I, Würch A, Kirschning CJ, Wagner H, Wallich R, Lamers

MC, Simon MM. Direct Toll-like receptor 2 mediated co-stimulation of T cells in the mouse system as a basis for chronic inflammatory joint disease. Arthritis Res Ther. 2004;6(5):R433-46. Epub 2004 Jul 19. PMID:15380043

Sood SK ed. Lyme Borreliosis in Europe and North America: Epidemiology and Clinical Practice. Hoboken New Jersey: Wiley and Sons, Inc., 2011.

Speelman P, de Jongh BM, Wolfs TF, Wittenberg J; Kwaliteitsinstituut voor de

Gezondheidszorg (CBO). [Guideline 'Lyme borreliosis'].[Article in Dutch]. Ned Tijdschr Geneeskd. 2004 Apr 3;148(14):659-63. PMID:15106316

Sréter T, Sréterné Lancz Z, Széll Z, Egyed L. [Rickettsia helvetica: an emerging tick-borne pathogen in Hungary and Europe]. [Article in Hungarian]. Orv Hetil. 2005 Dec 11;146(50):2547-52. PMID:16440500

Steere AC. Musculoskeletal manifestations of Lyme disease. Am J Med. 1995 Apr 24;98(4A):44S-48S; discussion 48S-51S. Review.

Steere AC, Bartenhagen NH, Craft JE, Hutchinson GJ, Newman JH, Rahn DW, Sigal LH, Spieler PN, Stenn KS, Malawista SE. The early clinical manifestations of Lyme disease. Ann Intern Med. 1983 Jul;99(1):76-82.

Steere AC, Berardi VP, Weeks KE, Logigian EL, Ackermann R. Evaluation of the intrathecal antibody response to Borrelia burgdorferi as a diagnostic test for Lyme neuroborreliosis. J Infect Dis. 1990 Jun;161(6):1203-9.

Steere AC, Gibofsky A, Patarroyo ME, Winchester RJ, Hardin JA, Malawista SE. Chronic Lyme arthritis. Clinical and immunogenetic differentiation from rheumatoid arthritis. Ann Intern Med. 1979 Jun;90(6):896-901.

Steere AC, Malawista SE, Bartenhagen NH, Spieler PN, Newman JH, Rahn DW, Hutchinson GJ, Green J, Snydman DR, Taylor E. The clinical spectrum and treatment of Lyme disease. Yale J Biol Med. 1984 Jul-Aug;57(4):453-61.

Steere AC, Sikand VK. The presenting manifestations of Lyme disease and the outcomes of treatment. N Engl J Med. 2003 Jun 12;348(24):2472-4.

Sterman AB, Nelson S, Barclay P. Demyelinating neuropathy accompanying Lyme disease. Neurology 1982 Nov;32(11):1302-5.

Storch A, Vladimirtsev VA, Tumani H, Wellinghausen N, Haas A, Krivoshapkin VG, Ludolph AC. Viliuisk encephalomyelitis in Northeastern Siberia is not caused by Borrelia burgdorferi infection. Neurol Sci. 2008 Feb;29(1):11-4. Epub 2008 Apr 1. PMID:18379734

Stricker RB. Counterpoint: long-term antibiotic therapy improves persistent symptoms associated with lyme disease. Clin Infect Dis. 2007 Jul 15;45(2):149-57. Epub 2007 Jun 5. PMID:17578772

Stricker RB, Johnson L. Lyme disease: a turning point. Expert Rev Anti Infect Ther. 2007 Oct;5(5):759-62. PMID:17914908

Stricker RB, Johnson L. Chronic Lyme disease and the 'Axis of Evil'. Future Microbiol. 2008 Dec;3(6):621-4. PMID:19072179

Stricker RB, Johnson L. Gender bias in chronic lyme disease. J Womens Health (Larchmt). 2009 Oct;18(10):1717-8; author reply 1719-20. PMID:19857097

Stricker RB, Johnson L. Lyme disease diagnosis and treatment: lessons from the AIDS epidemic. Minerva Med. 2010 Dec;101(6):419-25. PMID: 21196901

Stricker RB, Johnson L. Lyme disease: the next decade. Infect Drug Resist. 2011;4:1-9. Epub 2011 Jan 7. PMID:21694904

Stricker RB, Lautin A, Burrascano JJ. Lyme disease: point/
counterpoint. Expert Rev Anti Infect Ther. 2005 Apr;3(2):155-65.
PMID:15918774

Stricker RB, Savely VR, Motanya NC, Giclas PC. Complement split
products c3a and c4a in chronic lyme disease. Scand J Immunol. 2009
Jan;69(1):64-9. PMID:19140878

Summers BA, Straubinger AF, Jacobson RH, Chang YF, Appel
MJ, Straubinger RK. Histopathological studies of experimental
lyme disease in the dog. J Comp Pathol. 2005 Jul;133(1):1-13.
PMID:15904927

Tauber SC, Ribes S, Ebert S, Heinz T, Fingerle V, Bunkowski
S, Kugelstadt D, Spreer A, Jahn O, Eiffert H, Nau R. Long-term
intrathecal infusion of outer surface protein C from Borrelia
burgdorferi causes axonal damage. J Neuropathol Exp Neurol. 2011
Sep;70(9):748-57. PMID:21865883

Taylor RS, Simpson IN. Review of treatment options for lyme
borreliosis. J Chemother. 2005 Sep;17 Suppl 2:3-16. PMID:16315580

Telford SR III, Wormser GP. Bartonella spp. transmission by ticks not
established. Emerg Infect Dis. 2010 Mar;16(3):379-84.

Tory HO, Zurakowski D, Sundel RP. Outcomes of children treated for
Lyme arthritis: results of a large pediatric cohort. J Rheumatol. 2010
May;37(5):1049-55. Epub 2010 Apr 1. PMID:20360182

Treib J, Woessner R, Dobler G, Fernandez A, Hozler G, Schimrigk K.
Clinical value of specific intrathecal production of antibodies. Acta
virol 1997 Feb;41(1):27-30.

Tuuminen T, Hedman K, Söderlund-Venermo M, Seppälä I. Acute
parvovirus B19 infection causes nonspecificity frequently in Borrelia
and less often in Salmonella and Campylobacter serology, posing a
problem in diagnosis of infectious arthropathy. Clin Vaccine Immunol.
2011 Jan;18(1):167-72. Epub 2010 Nov 24. PMID:21106777

Vel'gin SO, Protas II, Ponomarev VV, Drakina SA, Shcherba VV. [Clinical polymorphism of neuroborreliosis at a late stage of the disease].[Article in Russian]. Zh Nevrol Psikhiatr Im S S Korsakova. 2006;106(3):48-51. PMID:16608111

Vojdani A. Antibodies as predictors of complex autoimmune diseases and cancer. Int J Immunopathol Pharmacol. 2008 Jul-Sep;21(3):553-66. Erratum in Int J Immunopathol Pharmacol. 2008 Oct-Dec;21(4):following 1051. PMID:18831922

Volkman DJ. An appraisal of "chronic Lyme disease". N Engl J Med. 2008 Jan 24;358(4):429; author reply 430-1. PMID:18219750

Wagner V, Zima E, Geller L, Merkely B. [Acute atrioventricular block in chronic Lyme disease].[Article in Hungarian]. Orv Hetil. 2010 Sep 26;151(39):1585-90. PMID:20840915

Wahlberg P, Nyman D. [Chronic Lyme borreliosis--fact or fiction?]. [Article in Finnish]. Duodecim. 2009;125(12):1269-76. PMID:19711595

WebMD. Lyme Disease Symptoms. http://arthritis.webmd.com/tc/lyme-disease-symptoms

Weintraub P. Cure Unknown: Inside the Lyme Epidemic. New York:Saint Martin's Griffin, 2009.

Weissenbacher S, Ring J, Hofmann H. Gabapentin for the symptomatic treatment of chronic neuropathic pain in patients with late-stage lyme borreliosis: a pilot study. Dermatology. 2005;211(2):123-7. PMID:16088158

Weissmann G. "Chronic Lyme" and other medically unexplained syndromes. FASEB J. 2007 Feb;21(2):299-301. PMID:17267382

Widhe M, Jarefors S, Ekerfelt C, Vrethem M, Bergstrom S, Forsberg P, Ernerudh J. Borrelia-specific interferon-gamma and interleukin-4 secretion in cerebrospinal fluid and blood during Lyme borreliosis in humans: association with clinical outcome. J Infect Dis. 2004 May 15;189(10):1881-91. Epub 2004 Apr 26. PMID:15122525

Wielgat P, Pancewicz S, Hermanowska-Szpakowicz T, Kondrusik M, Zajkowska J, Grygorczuk S, Popko J, Zwierz K. [Activity of lysosomal exoglycosidases in serum of patients with chronic borrelia arthritis].[Article in Polish]. Przegl Epidemiol. 2004;58(3):451-8. PMID:15730009

Wormser GP. Treatment and prevention of Lyme disease, with emphasis on antimicrobial therapy for neuroborreliosis and vaccination. Semin Neurol. 1997 Mar;17(1):45-52. Review.

Wormser GP, Schwartz I. Antibiotic treatment of animals infected with Borrelia burgdorferi. Clin Microbiol Rev. 2009 Jul;22(3):387-95. PMID:19597005

Wormser GP, Shapiro ED. Implications of gender in chronic Lyme disease. J Womens Health (Larchmt). 2009 Jun;18(6):831-4. PMID:19514824

Zajkowska J, Czupryna P, Pancewicz SA, Kondrusik M, Moniuszko A. Acrodermatitis chronica atrophicans. Lancet Infect Dis. 2011 Oct;11(10):800. PMID:21958583

Zajkowska JM, Kondrusik M, Pancewicz SA, Grygorczuk S, Jamiołkowski J, Stalewska J. [Comparison of test with antigen VlsE (C6) with tests with recombinant antigens in patients with Lyme borreliosis].[Article in Polish]. Pol Merkur Lekarski. 2007 Aug;23(134):95-9. PMID:18044336

Zajkowska JM, Swierzbińska R, Pancewicz SA, Kondrusik M, Hermanowska-Szpakowicz T. [Concentration of soluble CD4, CD8, CD25 receptors as well IFN-gamma and IL-4 released by lymphocyte of chronic Lyme patients cultured with 3 genotypes of Borrelia burgdorferi].[Article in Polish]. Pol Merkur Lekarski. 2004 May;16(95):447-50. PMID:15518424

Zalaudek I, Leinweber B, Kerl H, Müllegger RR. Acrodermatitis chronica atrophicans in a 15-year-old girl misdiagnosed as venous insufficiency for 6 years. 173. J Am Acad Dermatol. 2005 Jun;52(6):1091-4. PMID:15928636

Zeaiter Z, Liang Z, Raoult D. Genetic classification and differentiation of Bartonella species based on comparison of partial ftsZ gene sequences. J Clin Microbiol. 2002 Oct;40(10):3641-7. PMID:12354859

Zu-Rhein GM, Lo SC, Hulette CM, Powers JM. A novel cerebral microangiopathy with endothelial cell atypia and multifocal white matter lesions: a direct mycoplasmal infection? J Neuropathol Exp Neurol. 2007 Dec;66(12):1100-17. PMID:18090919

Dr. Schaller has been published in:

Journal of the American Medical Association

Journal of Clinical Neuroscience

Medscape (Academic Journal of WebMD)

Journal of the American Society of Child and Adolescent Psychiatry

American Journal of Psychiatry

European Journal of Child and Adolescent Psychiatry

Compounding Pharmaceuticals: Triad

Fleming Revell Press (Four Languages)

Internal Medicine News

Family Practice News

Spire Mass Market Books

Internet Journal of Family Medicine

Greenwood Press

Child and Adolescent Psychiatry Drug Alerts

Hope Academic Press

Clinical Psychiatry News

Psychiatric Drug Alerts

Townsend Journal

OB/GYN News

AMA News

Currents

A Sample of Other Books by Dr. Schaller

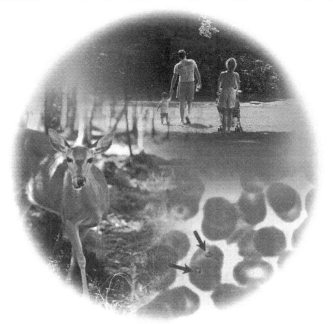

JAMES SCHALLER, M.D.

The Diagnosis and Treatment of

Babesia

Lyme's Cruel Cousin: the OTHER Tick-borne Infection

This large textbook is clear and easy to read. It is really three books. While some points are partially outdated since 2006, much would be considered new to most readers.

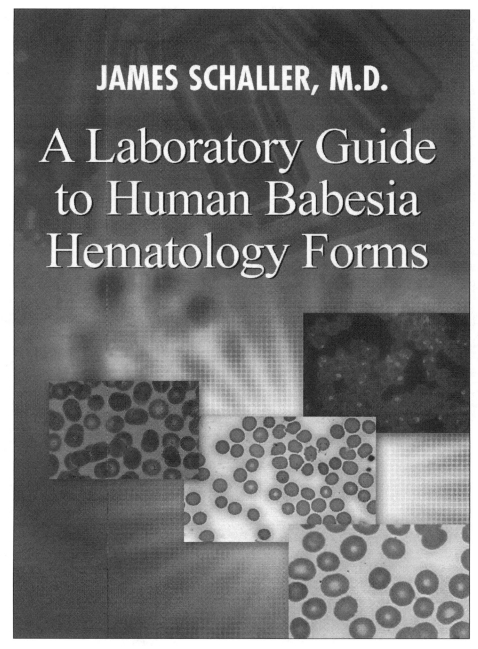

JAMES SCHALLER, M.D.

A Laboratory Guide to Human Babesia Hematology Forms

The Only Hematology Book Exclusively Dedicated to Babesia.

Artemisinin, Artesunate, Artemisinic Acid and Other Derivatives of Artemisia Used for Malaria, Babesia and Cancer

A Health Care Practitioner's Guide to Dosage, Side Effects, Effectiveness, Toxicity and Interactions. A Review of the Research on the Most Common Clinical Artemisia Medications.

JAMES SCHALLER, M.D.

The Most Up-To-Date Academic and Patient-Centered Book on Practical Artemisia Babesia Issues.

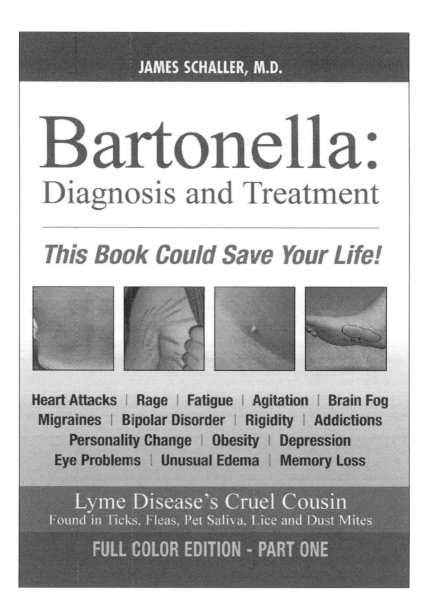

Bartonella diagnosis is very complex. This current text creatively used a new set of tools based on solid research of blood vessel and skin augmentation chemicals created by Bartonella. It literally creates a full Bartonella physical exam. This book helps with limited basic lab testing, and prevents the use of routinely relapsing or poor treatments promoted in both traditional and integrative medicine. No other book on this topic is based on over a thousand top research articles, and no one had published anything remotely close to replacing this work in over five years.

When Traditional Medicine Fails...

YOUR GUIDE TO
MOLD TOXINS

Gary Rosen, Ph.D. & James Schaller, M.D.

- **WHAT THEY ARE**
- **WHO THEY HURT**
- **AND WHAT YOU CAN
  DO TO RECLAIM YOUR CHILD'S HEALTH,
  LEARNING AND BEHAVIOR**

Includes Home Detox Program

Dr. Schaller is a Certified Mold Investigator
and a Certified Mold Remediator. Here is Another Practical
and Readable Mold Mycotoxin Book.

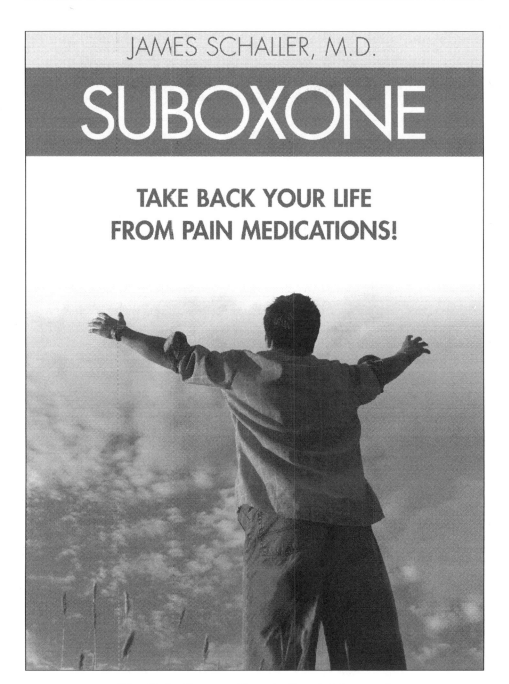

The Only Current, Practical and Advanced
Clinical Book on this Revolutionary Treatment for
Opioid Addiction and Modest Pain.

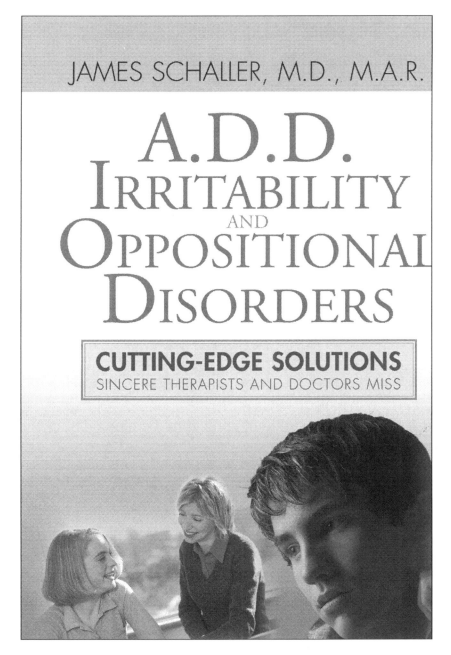

The many missed medical and neurological causes of poor focus and bad behaviors can no longer be ignored. This unique text advances medicine and shows how much in youth psychiatry has medical roots that are ignored or unknown even in solid child and adolescent psychiatry practices.

Disclaimer

Dr. Schaller is not a specialist in infectious disease medicine. He is also not a pathologist. Both of these specialties have over 2,000 diseases to treat and study. Dr. Schaller is only interested in four infections and has read and published on only these four. The medical ideas, health thoughts, health comments, products and any claims made about specific illnesses, diseases, and causes of health problems in this book are purely speculative, hypothetical, and are not meant to be authoritative in any setting. No comment or image has been evaluated by the FDA, CDC, NIH, IDSA or the AMA. Never assume any United States medical body, society, or the majority of American physicians endorse any comment in this book. No comment in this book is approved by any government agency, medical body or medical society. Nothing in this book is to be used to diagnose, treat, cure or prevent disease. The information provided in this book is for educational purposes only. It is not intended as a substitute for the advice from your physician or other health care professionals. This book is not intended to replace or adjust any information contained on, or in, any product label or packaging.

No patient should use the information in this book for the diagnosis or treatment of any health problem, or for prescription of any medication or other treatment. You should consult with a health care professional before deciding on any diagnosis, or initiating any treatment plan of any kind. Dr. Schaller does not claim to be an expert in any illness, disease or treatment. In this book, he is merely sharing one of his interests. Please do not start any diet, exercise or supplementation program, or take any type of nutrient, herb, or medication, without clear consultation with your licensed health care provider.

Babesia or Bartonella diagnosis or treatment comments and reports of possible positive or negative treatment outcomes are hypothetical. No treatment should be rejected or embraced by anyone, based on the preliminary research and study in this book.

In this book, Dr. Schaller makes no authoritative or proven claim about any diagnosis, lab testing or treatment. Dr. Schaller only offers hypothetical ideas. Dr. Schaller makes no authoritative claims about medications, nutrients, herbs or various types of alternative medicine.

The ideas in this book will need to be submitted to your local expert in allopathic, osteopathic or progressive medicine, or to other licensed health care practitioners. This book is not meant to be an informal or formal guideline book that presumes to control 800,000 physicians, or the 300 million patients they serve. You are asked to let the wisdom of your health care practitioners, and your own study, be a starting point to guide treatment tailored specifically to your body. Again, Dr. Schaller makes no claim to be an expert in any aspect of medicine. He makes no claim to know more than other physicians.

Additionally, Dr. Schaller makes no claim that any statement in this book is correct.

Since this appears to be the first book exclusively dedicated to advanced modern cutting-edge tick and flea infection expanded diagnosis criteria, it is very likely to contain errors This is common with books that are the first on such sensitive topics. Every reasonable effort has been made not to try to overstate findings. Further, it is important to realize that any single lab finding or treatment outcome can have multiple causes, and not all of these may be known to this author, or to other health practitioners. Therefore, all health care practitioners should look for other confirmations outside this book before beginning on any treatment plan, if possible.

Contacting Dr. Schaller

Should you wish to talk to Dr. Schaller he offers individualized education consults, which can be arranged by calling 239-263-0133. Please leave all your phone numbers, a working email and a fax number. These consults are typically in 15 minute units and can last as long as you wish. All that is required is the completion of a short informed consent form.

If you would like a full diagnostic consult or to see Dr. Schaller as a patient, know he treats patients from all over the USA and from outside the country. He meets with you first and then does follow-up care with you by phone. He does require you to have a family doctor, internist or pediatrician, since he is only a consultant.

If you would like to fly in to see Dr. Schaller, his staff are very familiar with all the closest airports, and we have special hotel discounts.

I wish you the very best health!

Warm Regards,
Rona C. MBA
Office Manager